MW00587208

TRIPPY

TRIPPY

The Peril and Promise of Medicinal Psychedelics

Ernesto Londoño

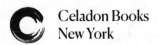

Celadon Books
New York

www.celadonbooks.com

Maps illustrated by Rich Tommaso

Library of Congress Cataloging-in-Publication Data

Names: Londoño, Ernesto, author.
Title: Trippy : the peril and promise of medicinal psychedelics / Ernesto Londoño.
Description: First edition. | New York : Celadon Books, 2024. | Includes
    bibliographical references and index.
Identifiers: LCCN 2023053304 | ISBN 9781250878540 (hardcover) | ISBN
    9781250878557 (ebook)
Subjects: LCSH: Hallucinogenic drugs. | Ayahuasca—Therapeutic use. |
    Hallucinogenic plants—Therapeutic use. | Hallucinogenic drugs and
    religious experience.
Classification: LCC RM324.8 .L66 2024 | DDC 615.7/883—dc23/eng/20240102
LC record available at https://lccn.loc.gov/2023053304

Our books may be purchased in bulk for promotional, educational, or business use. Please contact your local bookseller or the Macmillan Corporate and Premium Sales Department at 1-800-221-7945, extension 5442, or by email at MacmillanSpecialMarkets@macmillan.com.

First Edition: 2024

10 9 8 7 6 5 4 3 2 1

To the memory of my late grandparents
Hernando Martínez and Natalia Jaramillo, whose grit
and melancholy live within me

CONTENTS

TRIPPY

PREFACE

ROBERT FITZGERALD WALKED INTO A spacious house in a quiet Austin neighborhood for a three-day blitz of psychedelic therapy knowing very little about what lay ahead.

The army veteran, a politically conservative father of three, had no clue that the treatment center, All Tribes Medicine Assembly, was technically a church. He had heard next to nothing about Whitney Lasseter, a self-professed "sorceress of light," who had created the church a few months earlier to support some claim to legal protection for her psychedelic treatment practice.

Robert did not know that Whitney was a former drug addict and stripper who spent much of her adult life cycling in and out of rehab, until stumbling across a drug she credits with saving her life and instilling a sense of purpose. The weary and beleaguered people who sign up for her three-day retreats are subjected to a jolting protocol that includes an Amazonian ritual that leaves burn marks on the skin, a dose of psychedelic mushrooms so large it is dubbed "heroic," and smoking a toad venom that obliterates a person's consciousness within seconds.

Robert had given no thought to whether any of what he was about to do was legal.

What the thirty-five-year-old knew for sure on that day in late October 2022 was that a long spiral of depression had left him suicidal, in urgent need of help—and that the mainstream mental health care system had failed him.

Antidepressants made him feel like a zombie. Therapists he saw at the Department of Veterans Affairs struck Robert as unhelpful and rote, as though they were all reading from the same script. His most recent taste of conventional medicine, a haunting, humiliating two-day stay in the psychiatric ward, sapped what remained of his faith in the health care system.

Two weeks after a suicide attempt, Robert put himself in Whitney's care as a Hail Mary of sorts.

A little over a year before, working alongside veteran friends, he had become deeply invested in helping Afghans flee their country amid the chaotic American withdrawal that left the Taliban in control of Kabul. As a monumentally frustrating and all-encompassing effort came to an end, Robert began noticing vague, intrusive thoughts about death. They seemed to convey that he wouldn't be around much longer and were sometimes accompanied by visions of a fiery car crash.

Over time, those dark thoughts hardened, convincing Robert that his wife and three young kids would be better off without him. One morning in mid-October 2022, after drinking half a bottle of vodka, he drove to a park near his suburban house in Pennsylvania, stuck the barrel of a pistol inside his mouth, and tried to muster the will to end it all.

"My mom was calling, my sister was calling, and my wife was calling," he told me. "I wouldn't answer any phone calls, because I'm just sitting there, trying so hard to pull the trigger."

Sensing her son was deeply unwell, Robert's mother kept calling until he answered. That frantic conversation triggered an intervention.

She called the police, who soon found Robert, took his weapon, and drove him to a hospital, where he was placed on a suicide watch.

"Everything became exposed, and I was no longer alone with these thoughts, alone with everything," Robert said. "I realized how much I needed help."

In the blurry days that followed, other veterans who had also come close to putting a bullet through their brains told him about Whitney and the astonishing turnarounds they had experienced after taking psychedelics under her care.

Figuring he had little to lose, Robert wired the $2,888 retreat fee and booked a flight to Austin.

〰 It may seem befuddling that Robert and his family saw fit to put his perturbed mind in the hands of someone like Whitney. Yet lives like theirs are frequently intersecting as more people who have lost faith in conventional medicine are drawn to the booming, largely unregulated field of medicinal psychedelics.

Often, the most desperate wind up being treated by practitioners who aren't waiting around for a clear regulatory framework or a more robust scientific understanding of the promise and perils of these drugs. They are being treated by the biggest risk-takers.

Whitney has come to believe the war on drugs should have been declared a lost cause a long time ago. And she is among a growing field of psychedelic practitioners who are taking a crusading spirit to undermine the case for prohibition, one patient at a time.

"These medicines shouldn't be restricted," Whitney told me. "They are our birthright."

In 2021, at least 48,183 people killed themselves in the United States, according to the Centers for Disease Control and Prevention, which noted that a significant rise in younger people ending their lives has pushed the nation's suicide rate to a near record high. To put it into perspective, that figure is more than double the estimated 22,900 murders the Federal Bureau of Investigation recorded that same year.

Twenty-four percent of Americans described their mental health as fair or poor in 2022, a record high, according to a Gallup poll. Among people between the ages of eighteen and thirty-four, the percentage was 46 percent. A broad majority of Americans report feeling deeply frustrated with the mental health care system. The cost of therapy is out of reach for many, and even those with means often struggle to find timely care. Antidepressants, which were hailed as a revolutionary tool in psychiatry when they became widely available in the 1980s, have loud detractors who point to their uneven efficacy and serious side effects, including emotional blunting and sexual dysfunction.

These shortcomings have become a bonanza for champions of the curative power of psychedelics. The rapidly growing and strikingly diverse community includes well-respected scientists, religious leaders, new age hippies, and veterans, as well as Indigenous healers who regard psychoactive plants as sacred conduits to spiritual realms.

The journalist Michael Pollan turbocharged their ambitions in 2018 with *How to Change Your Mind*. The bestselling book recounts how a promising wave of research into psychedelics was abandoned abruptly after President Richard Nixon declared the war on drugs in the 1970s. Pollan spotlighted key people working to bring a shadowy field into the mainstream, a shift that has accelerated at dizzying speed since then.

Regulators at the Food and Drug Administration have designated MDMA, the drug known as ecstasy, and psilocybin, the psychoactive compound in psychedelic mushrooms, as "breakthrough therapies." That label means the two drugs, which have been used in clinical trials to treat patients with post-traumatic stress disorder and severe depression, may offer substantial improvements over existing therapies. Both are widely expected to get FDA approval for mainstream clinical use by 2024.

The Department of Veterans Affairs has begun administering psychedelics to some veterans as part of clinical trials designed to assess their potential to treat PTSD and substance abuse. The federal government in 2021 began to fund research into the therapeutic potential of psychedelics for the first time in half a century.

Dr. Joshua Gordon, the director of the National Institute of Mental Health, a federal agency, said that the most remarkable feature of these drugs is how quickly they relieve symptoms and how long their effects last for many patients. "The drugs have remarkable potential," he said in an interview. "If they work as well in larger studies as early results would suggest, these are going to be important elements in our arsenal."

The theory at the heart of this research is that psychedelics can induce quick and profound changes in mood and outlook, seemingly by stimulating key receptors in the brain. Scientists theorize that by disrupting routine patterns of thought and memory processing, psychedelic trips often yield profound insights and a reprieve from the obsessive thought loops often associated with mental illness.

Anticipating how disruptive those drugs could be in mental health care, hundreds of clinicians have undergone formal training to become psychedelic-assisted therapists. Many have begun getting real-world experience at ketamine clinics, where people with depression are given off-label infusions of the anesthetic, which, at low doses, produces a dissociative psychedelic experience.

Since 2019, venture capitalists have provided seed funding for dozens of publicly traded psychedelic biotech companies. Several of those have filed a flurry of patent applications in an effort to dominate a corner of an industry that promises to make fortunes.

This sector of the field, which is in its infancy, has much to learn from the sprawling psychedelic retreat industry in Latin America, which has roots in ancient Indigenous rituals. Each year, thousands travel to Brazil, Peru, Mexico, and Costa Rica for psychedelic treatment at facilities that range from backpacker basic to decadent luxury. Some blend ayahuasca with meditation training. One of the most expensive ones, which promises a "shortcut to happiness," charges upward of $7,000 for a week.

Elected officials have taken note of the broadening appeal of drugs that were long associated with hippies and the counterculture movement. A handful of states and cities have decriminalized the use of certain psychedelics. Voters in Oregon in 2020 approved a first-of-its-kind measure that regulates the therapeutic use of psilocybin. Between 2017 and 2022, lawmakers have introduced at least seventy-four bills seeking to expand research into, or access to, psychedelics.

A study published in the *Journal of the American Medical Association* predicts that if psychedelics follow the political trajectory of cannabis, a majority of states will legalize psychedelics by the 2030s.

While it may seem that psychedelic therapy has become increasingly available, for people in crisis like Robert, spiritual retreats remain the most accessible entry point. It's a realm where practitioners have begun to operate with a striking degree of audacity, understanding that administering and selling psychedelics could lead to felony charges.

"I am willing to take the risk because I know I'm doing good work," Whitney told me. "I've seen lives change, and I'm willing to be a martyr for the cause."

Whitney told me she has found working with veterans particularly rewarding because they tend to be highly motivated, disciplined, and trained to follow instructions. But there's also a pragmatic reason Whitney decided to link her brand to the veteran mental health care crisis: she thinks it makes her less likely to face scrutiny from law enforcement. "What are they going to do, bust in here and say I'm not doing good work?" she said. "I have men here who have protected them and been willing to sacrifice their lives for their country."

〰〰 Robert's retreat was hastily put together. Whitney had been planning a Halloween extravaganza at the church and was preparing for a trip to Egypt. But when she heard that there was an army veteran in crisis, a guy who had a pistol in his mouth just days earlier, Whitney cleared her schedule for three days.

Shortly before the first ceremony of the retreat, Whitney gathered the five participants in the living room of the house, which had been reconfigured as a ceremonial space with a large golden Buddha statue, a large mandala, and a cross. Whitney handed each participant a vial of rosemary oil, telling them the scent helped bring repressed memories to the fore. To set their intention for the days ahead, she instructed the participants to draw three concentric circles on a blank page of their journal and sketch a cross over them, making a bull's-eye. On the small inside circle, Whitney told them to write a simple phrase summarizing the desired end state. In the second layer of quadrants, she told them to jot down thoughts on what it would take to accomplish that. On the outer quadrants, Whitney asked them to imagine how that state would make them feel. The intentions needed to be framed in positive terms—appealing for a state of joy, for instance, rather than wishing away anger.

Then, she said, they needed to trust that what they wanted was within reach, but not get too fixated on how it would materialize. "Anything you desire can be yours," Whitney said. "Look for signs that it's arriving."

Robert followed her instructions dutifully. In the center of his design were three words: *freedom, joy,* and *stability*.

Soon, Whitney produced the first set of "medicines" for the retreat. The patients would be given rapé, a tobacco snuff from the Amazon that is blown into a person's nostrils, producing an intense head rush. Then a squirt from the sananga plant, which Indigenous people in the Amazon use to sharpen their vision and instincts, would be dropped in their eyes. Finally, each would get burn marks on their forearm to administer kambo, the toad venom. The three medicines would be uncomfortable—distressing, even—Dani Amelio, a Reiki practitioner who co-facilitated the retreat, told the wary participants in a warm voice. Buckets for vomit were placed by each person's mat.

"It's going to be burning up what's been harbored in the depths of your being," Dani said. "It's going to be brought up to be released and let go."

It was important—vital—to trust the medicine, Dani said, to surrender to the process completely. "Allow the medicine to just do what the medicine does," she advised. "Communicate with the medicine," she said. "Thank the medicine, even before we put it on. Do a little blessing on the medicine, and just show reverence to the medicine."

With gentle music playing in the background, she flicked a lighter on and set the tip of a stick on fire. Tenderly, she pressed the stick on each person's arm and readied the venom.

Had I watched this scene a few years ago, chances are that I would have been deeply alarmed. I may have run outside, refusing to be complicit, even as a bystander, in what was about to happen. But instead, I took deep breaths and prayed that Whitney and Dani knew what they were doing. In the eyes of the participants, at once weary and hopeful, I recognized a familiar state of surrender. After all, not too long ago, I was in their shoes, taking a massive leap of faith.

1

IN BRAZIL, AN UNRAVELING AND AN OFF-RAMP

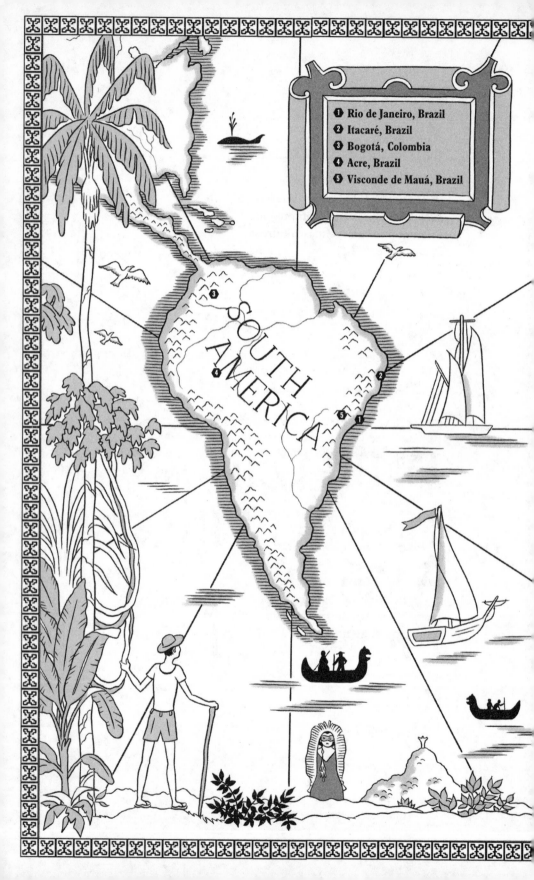

1. Rio de Janeiro, Brazil
2. Itacaré, Brazil
3. Bogotá, Colombia
4. Acre, Brazil
5. Visconde de Mauá, Brazil

SOUTH AMERICA

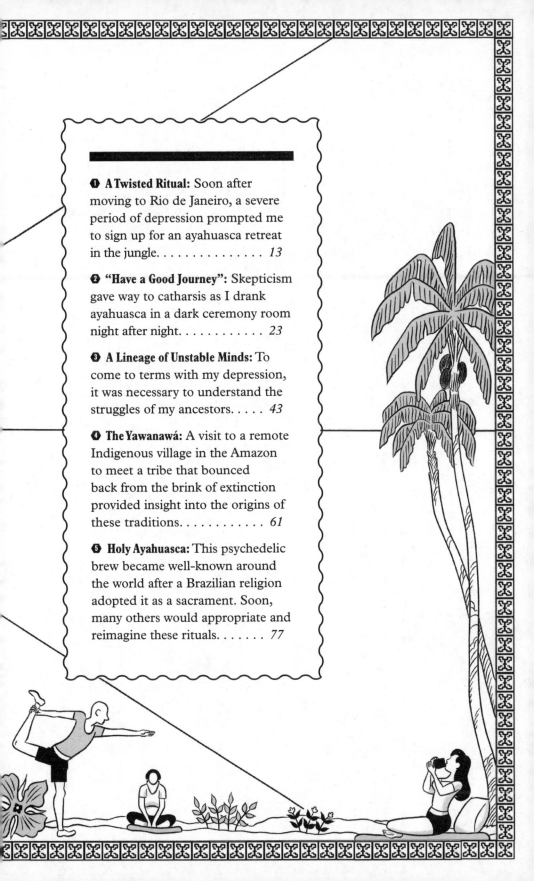

1 A TWISTED RITUAL

IF I HAD TO PUT a marker on the low point, it would be the warm, breezy November night when I lost my balance—and nearly lost my life.

Standing on the ledge of the terrace in my apartment in Rio de Janeiro, overlooking the waves that soothe the edges of the frenetic city, I struck the dancer's pose—again. The yoga move had become a twisted depression ritual: Clasping my right ankle with my right hand, I would thrust that leg into the air, toes pointing skyward. Left knee firmly locked, I gently lowered my torso toward the winding road twenty-one stories below and extended my left arm toward the horizon. Breathing deeply, I watched the flow of headlights light up and darken the pavement.

It had taken me years to master the pose. The trick is to keep the standing leg ramrod straight, which is harder than you'd think. If the knee wobbles, the stance collapses, and you tumble down, often headfirst. I began striking it regularly on the rim of the terrace because the strength and focus it demands had a way of quieting my mind, which had become unbearably restless in the weeks following my move to Brazil in mid-2017.

As depression mounted and sleepless nights gave way to angst-ridden days, what had been a soothing ritual became a manifestation of the suicidal ideation swelling within me. Abstract thoughts about ending my life had become disconcertingly crisp. Suddenly, there were the outlines of what a plan might entail, consideration given to how much effort various means would require, and an inclination, always, toward endings that would appear accidental.

That evening, as my chest dipped over the edge, my knee wobbled. A ripple of vertigo coursed down my spine, and I fell sideways. For a moment, I couldn't decide whether I felt lucky or defeated. Then, an unexpected thought—an instruction, really—seeped into my mind. I was to adopt a dog—imminently. I had been tempted to do so ever since I stumbled into a dog adoption event at a park in Copacabana while running during my first week in Rio. I had fallen madly in love with a traumatized, caramel-colored mutt with a crooked mouth and a couple of scars on his ears. After holding him for half an hour, feeling his heart pound like a drum, I walked away. Depression has a way of drowning even the best intentions in a pond of ambivalence. After my downfall, even in the midst of the fog that dulled my mind at the time, this much became clear: being responsible for another living being would nix this flirtation with death. A dog's bulging bladder would get me out of bed in the morning, which had become a growing struggle. And being greeted by the crackling excitement of a pet reunited with his human might make my sparsely furnished apartment feel a bit more like a home.

〰〰 This creeping despair was not how I imagined I would settle into one of the most coveted jobs in American journalism: the *New York Times* Brazil bureau chief.

Brazil is a land of lush beauty, where jagged hills sprout out of the ocean in majestic disarray. The music can break and mend your heart in the same stanza. The laid-back and improvisational approach to life appealed to me after the frenzy of New York City.

But the job also came with a warning: Brazil is not for beginners—a saying shared knowingly by expats who love to hate and hate to love the notoriously indecipherable nation of 218 million. The threat of violence seems to lurk permanently in the air, keeping the senses sharp and adrenaline pumping. Then there's the bureaucracy, so absurd that it can only be appreciated as theater.

I shrugged off the admonitions. After all, I was born and raised in Colombia in the 1980s and 1990s, turbulent years of drug trade–fueled armed conflict. I spent the better part of my twenties bouncing between Iraq and Afghanistan as a correspondent for the *Washington Post*.

The assignment was to cover the southern half of South America, five countries known for succulent steaks, mouthwatering Malbecs, and beautiful men. I'd get to sit down with heads of state and celebrities, traverse the Amazon rainforest by boat, and spend nights scanning the majestic sky over Chile's northern desert, counting shooting stars. With a generous expense account, I'd be limited only by creative wherewithal. Accepting the position felt like winning the journalism lottery.

〰〰 Just weeks after arriving and signing a lease for a penthouse unit with a private pool and within walking distance of the beach, I began to spiral into a sinkhole of despondency. Each new day felt more agonizing than the last. I fought insomnia with increasingly generous pours of single malt whiskey, which induced a restless form of sleep and left me feeling drained in the morning. Casual sex became my main prescription for a crippling sense of disconnection, but hooking up with strangers only deepened my isolation.

I had been prone to melancholy since childhood and had experienced bouts of depression before, but never one as intractable and paralyzing as this one. Depression ran in both sides of my bloodline, but I dwelled little on my genetic disposition to an illness that afflicts an estimated 280 million people globally. In keeping with a family tradition, I fought to keep my depression from spilling into public view. Because there was nothing wrong in my life that I could point to, my emotional state seemed incomprehensible, and the prospect of seeking professional help, unjustified. Besides, having covered war zones for years, I regarded my resilience as a core strength, a cornerstone of my personal and professional identity. I wasn't someone who asked for help.

〜〜 Booking one-way flights and packing my belongings into boxes every few years had become something of a way of life since I left Bogotá, my birthplace, in 1999 to attend college in the United States. I lingered in each new place long enough to get my heart broken a time or two, but always found an off-ramp before putting down the sort of roots that would make any place feel like home.

After graduating from college in 2003, I caught one lucky break after another in the cratering newspaper industry. At each stop, I sought to make myself indispensable and somehow weathered what seemed like an endless series of layoffs. Eventually, my career reached cruising altitude. After nine years at the *Washington Post*, the *Times* hired me in 2014 to join its editorial board, where I made an early splash with a series of editorials arguing in favor of normalizing diplomatic relations with Cuba.

Away from work, I had been dating John, a handsome public defender with sad eyes and a heart of gold, for a little over two years. We shared an apartment in the South Bronx with his rescue dog, Ham— short for Alexander Hamilton—a disheveled cairn terrier who went berserk with joy every evening when I walked through the door.

In early 2017, the international editors at the *Times* asked if I would be interested in the Brazil job. There was no compelling reason to put an end to my life in New York. But when the Brazil exit ramp appeared, I took it unblinkingly. These kinds of sharp turns had served me well professionally. To the extent that I pondered the trade-offs of a nomadic lifestyle, at each crossroads, I figured I was still young enough to ultimately lay down roots somewhere, find someone to come home to, and settle down—whatever that meant.

John seemed willing to join me. He flew to Rio about a month after I arrived for a trip that was meant to give us a chance to figure out how he might fit into my new life. But almost from the moment he walked in the door, we began arguing over petty things. I struggled to be anything other than cold and preoccupied in his presence. This man who had taken my breath away a couple of years back suddenly felt like a piece of clothing I had outgrown. It felt daunting to make room for him in this new life I was creating. As I'd done several times before, I was writing a new chapter that needed a clean slate and a brand-new cast of characters.

During John's visit, I worked long hours on my first few articles from the region, heeding the advice of an editor who said new correspondents needed to crack the front page and make a splash right out of the gate. I spent hours each day practicing Portuguese, a language whose similarity to my native Spanish gave me an edge on comprehension, but became disadvantageous when it came to trying to speak it. While I was consumed with work, John plunged head-on into Rio's hedonistic nightlife, once coming back home so drunk I found him asleep on the bathroom floor.

A week before he was scheduled to fly home, I broke up with him at a tapas restaurant with a sea view. It was a short and curt conversation in which we conveyed more with rigid body language than words.

〰 Rio would seem to be the ideal city for a newly single gay man. But as I set out to date, I got ghosted and stood up with striking frequency. I took these slights personally until I realized people from Rio are notoriously noncommittal and fickle when it comes to sticking to plans. Lots of people were friendly toward me as I got settled in, but it became apparent that many were mainly interested in freelance work at the *Times* or to persuade me to write about their work or causes. I grew increasingly distressed by the underside of my new hometown: the smell of raw sewage along the route from the airport;

the earsplitting music that soured trips to the beach; and the palpable sense of danger every time I left home. Rio was going through an extraordinarily violent period. Thronged beaches were often the target of mass robberies known as *arrastões*, in which swarms of young shirtless men moved in unison, wavelike, against their targets, snatching phones, backpacks, and wallets. Before going on one of the spectacular hikes around the city, I researched the route to find out whether tourists had been held up at knifepoint there in recent days.

Pouring myself into work had long been my default mode, and a reliable antidote to short-circuiting bouts of melancholy. Work always kept me afloat, it kept me on track, and it was the bedrock of my sense of self-worth. But during my early months in Brazil, I filed stories that sat for weeks without being edited, which made me feel like an asterisk on a map brimming with more urgent news unfolding elsewhere. I began feeling like a fraud, a sense that made it harder to focus on work.

At a hot yoga studio a few blocks from home, I often wept quietly as I practiced, my tears indistinguishable from sweat. While walking home, I stopped by a kiosk to buy a single cigarette, which I would light on my terrace as I took in the view and wondered how someone who seemingly had so much could feel so rotten.

Soon after my slip on the terrace, I went to SUIPA, the city's largest animal shelter, a teeming compound in a violent favela called Jacarezinho, where vets often treated animals struck by stray bullets. I handed an attendant a stack of profiles of dogs I had starred from those featured on its website. But as she brought them out one by one, I couldn't connect with any. One was missing a rear leg, and I felt gutted for turning her down and watching her being carried back to the jam-packed kennel, looking resigned. I was about to walk away when the shelter employee asked me to consider one last candidate that wasn't on the website. When she returned, my heart skipped a beat: she was carrying the traumatized dog I'd met in the park in Copacabana right after I landed. The white splotches on his belly and nose were unmistakable. I remembered his name, Hugo, and scrolled through my phone to show her the photos I had taken when I first considered bringing him home. Within minutes, I had signed all the forms required to take him home, and marveled at the serendipity.

Being responsible for Hugo did, in fact, force me to get out of bed in the morning. Rubbing his warm belly at night while he snored gently made me feel less lonely. His goofy face—he was unable to keep his long, sloppy tongue in his mouth—was one of the few things that made me smile. But he was not an antidepressant. While he imposed a tiny bit of structure on my life, I continued to languish. I slogged through workdays. I dreaded answering phone calls and found fault in every article I managed to get done. I feared it was a matter of time before it became apparent to colleagues that I was unwell—that I was not up to the task that had seemed like a dream come true just months before.

That was when the universe tossed me the loopiest of lifelines. It was shortly after Christmas 2017, which I spent alone in Rio. Howling winds rattled my windows. Sleep felt impossible. On a whim, I reached for my laptop and Googled "ayahuasca retreats in Brazil." It must have been close to 4:00 a.m.

I had been thinking of writing a piece about the growing popularity of ayahuasca retreats after a conversation with Dr. Jordan Sloshower, a Yale psychiatrist I met at my sister's engagement party shortly before moving to Brazil. Sloshower was among a new generation of psychiatrists dusting off research into the therapeutic potential of hallucinogens. The promising field had flourished in the 1950s and 1960s but had been hastily shut down when the compounds became illegal.

With a mop of unruly red hair, Sloshower looked more like a hippie living out of a van than an Ivy League shrink. His eyes widened with enthusiasm as he told me about all the people who were flocking to the Amazon to drink a powerful psychedelic brew. He had seen its potential to spark extraordinary transformations in people who were suffering. Clearly, this guy's interest in psychedelics was more than academic, I thought. Suddenly, my own interest became more than journalistic.

The first link I clicked led to a video that cast a spell on me. It featured Silvia Polivoy, the blue-eyed, silky-voiced founder of Spirit Vine Center, one of the first ayahuasca retreats catering to foreigners in Latin America, describing the mysterious healing modality she created in a lush strip of jungle near a northern Brazil beach town.

"With ayahuasca, we can see our patterns of behavior," explained Silvia, an Argentine psychotherapist who trained with Indigenous plant medicine experts. "Usually in our everyday life, we are so busy working, running, angry, whatever, we don't have the attention in the little things we do constantly."

The "tea," as she called it, could transform lives by producing vital insights that were hidden in plain sight. I was intrigued. Then the video got wacky. For ayahuasca to do its thing, Silvia said, participants needed to muster the courage to surrender.

"When they surrender, they go to another realm, where there's no more fear," she promised. "You can meditate, and suddenly, you will feel the oneness."

It all sounded bonkers. But Silvia's voice had a gentle conviction that reeled me in. Another realm. The end of fear. Ceremonies held at night in a jungle brimming with wildlife. Was I on the brink of joining a cult? Or was salvation at hand? What did I have to lose by gravitating toward this motherly woman and her jungle retreat? I snapped my laptop shut and slept better than I had in months.

〰〰 The following morning, I read the fine print. The nine-day retreat cost $2,550 and had some bizarre rules. Spirit Vine participants were served only vegetarian food. Weeks before arriving, retreatgoers were instructed to abstain from drinking alcohol and eating red meat, pork, and salty foods because "being clean prior to ceremony will facilitate a deeper process."

The last two rules were doozies. First, Silvia requested that participants abstain from having any kind of sex—including masturbating—for at least seven days prior to the retreat, during their time at Spirit Vine, and three days after leaving. The stated reason: "The process of orgasm itself expels a large amount of energy and opens up the energy field." And "going deeper into our personal journey," the website claimed, "requires an intact energy field."

Finally, Silvia asked participants to refrain from consuming news for at least one week prior to the retreat, warning that the news has "a deep effect on our mental and emotional state."

Instead of giving me pause, these directives only added to the allure of this strange place. A retreat application form asked prospective participants why they wanted to come. I wrote that I was eager to go "completely off the grid for a few days to focus on self-care and make time for introspection." There was a question about how well applicants can handle crises. I responded smugly: "Very well. I lived in war zones for several years, so I am calm and steady in times of crisis." Finally, applicants were asked to disclose any medical or psychological conditions. I noted that I took medicine for high blood pressure.

Silvia replied that afternoon, saying my application looked good except for the blood pressure drugs. "You have to ask your doctor for authorization to change this medication for something natural or another method," she said. "Blood pressure medication is not compatible with ayahuasca."

At the time, I was taking forty milligrams of quinapril every morning. I had first been prescribed the drug in my midtwenties by a doctor in Dallas who was mystified by my hypertension, given my youth and fitness level. The condition worsened over the years as I took on increasingly stressful jobs, leading a series of doctors to increase my dosage.

Had I been thinking straight as I was considering the Spirit Vine retreat, this would have been a deal-breaker. It's one thing to embark on an adventure of blue balls and culinary deprivation on the off chance that this mysterious tea would transport me to a realm without fear. But going off blood pressure medication to put my rambunctious mind through the psychedelic wringer was downright reckless. And yet, on some level, I had already crossed the Rubicon.

Nothing would stand in the way of getting my weary body to Silvia's jungle center. I emailed back a carefully worded reply assuring Silvia that I could keep my blood pressure in check by taking natural supplements and promised to bring a monitor to measure it before the ceremonies.

〰〰 That did the trick. I was in. With roughly a month to prepare for the retreat, I ate plenty of steak, drank heavily, and scanned the hookup apps, compensating for the days of privation that lay ahead. I slept with a listless flight attendant, a bouncy Israeli who was traveling the world after completing his military service, and a lanky Putin-loving Russian guy from Siberia. I walked away from each of these encounters feeling depleted and ashamed. But within hours, my eyes would be glued to the phone screen again, sending and receiving awkwardly posed naked photos—a ritual that raised a prospect of intimacy that seldom materialized. As the retreat date neared, I was forced to start the celibacy period early thanks to a sexually transmitted infection.

I didn't even attempt to abide by the no-news rule before the retreat. The city had been awash in violence during the 2018 Carnival, prompting the president to take drastic action and put the military in charge of restoring order in Rio de Janeiro. I was so frazzled while packing and preparing a story that I showed up at the wrong airport and missed my flight. Getting to the retreat in time required purchasing a new ticket for $400. After writing a hastily reported story during two short flights, I made it to Spirit Vine before sunset.

A sturdy gate that opened by remote control led down a road ringed by hibiscus shrubs with bright red and yellow flowers. As the gate snapped shut behind me, I had a momentary jolt of panic. My heart throbbed in my chest, a reminder that my body needed blood pressure medicine.

But there was no turning back.

2 "HAVE A GOOD JOURNEY"

THE FIRST PARTICIPANT I MET at Spirit Vine after dropping off my bag was Princess, a bubbly Texan with plump lips and thick braids. It turned out Princess was her real name, picked by a father whose country music career never quite took off. On a sweltering early afternoon in mid-February, the peak of Brazil's summer, we were floating on neon-colored noodles in the center's placid pond, surrounded by palm trees that looked like handheld fans and a chorus of frogs croaking in unison. Having filed a breaking story en route to the retreat, I was buzzing with discomfort from putting my phone on airplane mode for the next few days, when Princess asked the first of several unexpected questions I would get that week.

"Is this your first time with the medicine?" she wanted to know.

Taken aback by the euphemism, it took me a couple of beats to respond that, yes, I was an ayahuasca virgin.

Reading my body language, she asked if I was nervous. *Terrified* was closer to the truth, I confessed.

"You're *ready*," she assured me, seeming elated to have found a newbie. The medicine, Princess explained, draws people into the realm of sacred plants only when they're ready. The medicine knows what it's doing. *Trust* it.

A cult, I remember thinking again. *I have stumbled into a cult.*

The cult had paperwork, including a "hold harmless" agreement. After drying off, Princess and I joined the other participants in the main meeting room, an airy space with comfy daybeds arranged in a circle and decorated with psychedelic tapestries. That's where Silvia and her sidekick, a lanky guy named Rohan, who was maddeningly Zen and wore a perpetual smile, handed us forms. We were asked to list all medications we were taking, disclose past illicit drug use, and disclose whether we had ever attempted suicide. I truthfully divulged that my only brush with controlled substances had involved pot, which I smoked a handful of times and never particularly cared for; I left the suicide line blank. We had to agree not to sue Spirit Vine if something went terribly wrong with the medicine. After reading each page diligently, I certified that I was not currently suicidal and signed away my right to take legal action.

Once the forms were collected, Silvia and Rohan introduced themselves. Silvia had been trained as a psychotherapist in Buenos Aires, her hometown, which has among the highest rates of shrinks per capita in the world. She dabbled in hypnosis and other unconventional means to access childhood trauma until she read in a magazine about shamanic rituals in the Amazon. In the mid-1990s, she left her home and her practice to travel to Peru in search of Indigenous shamans who specialized in psychoactive plants.

Back then, finding ayahuasca communities required word-of-mouth referrals and major leaps of faith. Her first few ceremonies took place in jungle huts without running water, under the guidance of shamans who said little, spoke largely in metaphors, and blew thick fumes of tobacco into people's faces during rituals.

Silvia said she found more perplexity than enlightenment during the first few weeks she drank ayahuasca. Nearly a year into this self-imposed purgatory, she had a vision that would change her life. It involved a conversation with one of her late grandmothers, who Silvia says revealed how harrowing and traumatic her first years as an immigrant in Argentina had been.

One night after this revelation, Silvia had a vision that there was a slice of the jungle clamoring to be preserved. That image set her off on a journey across South America that ended early in the new millennium, when she set foot on the property in the Brazilian state of Bahia that would ultimately become Spirit Vine. She recognized it as the land that had reached out for help during that life-altering ayahuasca trip.

In 2004, she began hosting retreats on the land, becoming one of the pioneers of a psychedelic retreat industry that would see exponential growth in the years ahead as scores of other foreigners who found a toehold in the world of shamanism in the Amazon decided to appropriate and commodify sacred traditions.

Rohan, who is originally from India, had attended one of Silvia's early retreats. At the time, he worked as a software engineer at Amazon in Seattle, where he spent most of his waking hours high on pot. After a week in Silvia's care, he quit his job, gave up marijuana, and moved to Brazil to help run the weeklong retreats.

During our introductory session, Silvia addressed the group with grandmotherly warmth, but she made clear the center had strict rules and zero tolerance for rule breakers. Smoking was absolutely prohibited, and any cigarettes stashed away in suitcases needed to be turned over immediately. Any smuggled snacks would be seized and returned only at the end of the retreat because it was imperative that we stick to a sodium-free, plant-based diet. We were only to leave the property for authorized trips to a nearby beach every other day. There was a reminder about the sex abstinence rule, including masturbation.

With the rules out of the way, we went around the room introducing ourselves. There were three guys from Hungary who had traveled to Spirit Vine together. One had just learned his partner was expecting a baby, and he spent the retreat oscillating between feelings of joy and dread as he contemplated fatherhood.

A blond gay man from Germany, well acquainted with mind-altering drugs, brimmed with enthusiasm. He worked for a family of

Turkish billionaires, overseeing the upkeep of vacation homes scattered around the world. A skinny Polish woman who wore only black spent much of the retreat in tears as she dwelled on her dysfunctional relationship with her mom.

A middle-aged psychotherapist from the United Kingdom who had struggled with chronic pain her whole adult life claimed to have found the root cause during a ceremony: in a past life, she had been a Guatemalan peasant who went through life with an amputated leg.

When it was my turn to speak, I was surprised by the words that came out of my mouth after stating my name, country of origin, and profession.

"I feel like an instrument that hasn't been tuned in years," I said.

That night, before going to bed, I approached Silvia to let her know that I'd had no problem weaning myself off the blood pressure pills and that I was taking garlic supplements to keep it in check. In fact, my heartbeat had become audible at night since I stopped taking quinapril, and I could feel tiny bursts in the arteries in my neck as blood struggled to get to the brain. Silvia didn't seem interested in discussing my blood pressure. But she stared at me somewhat icily and offered an unwelcome observation.

"There's something you're repressing inside," she said. "Do you know what it might be?"

I muttered an avoidant response and walked away. I found her remark off-putting. I was not repressed. I was depressed.

〰〰 My annoyance with Silvia only grew the next day when we gathered around the center's meeting room, on spacious sofas, for our first workshop: Inner Child Integration. Silvia explained that much of our suffering is rooted in traumas endured during our early years. The goal of the session was to induce us to identify one such moment through a guided meditation. It could be anything—the first thing that popped into our minds—even if it felt random or inconsequential.

When we stumbled across an event, Silvia instructed us to have the adult version of ourselves comfort the ailing child, reaching across time to amend how that one consequential moment of our lives unfolded. We could embrace the child, shield it from abusers, or hold its hand, whatever felt right in the moment. Then we had to decide what action needed to be taken to undo the harm. We could confront an aggressor, remove the child from a dangerous environment, or call the police.

The whole thing insulted my intelligence. I refused to accept the premise that everyone had crippling, unresolved childhood trauma. The eagerness some of the participants showed in playing along made me want to scream. I was wondering if it was too late to walk away and ask for a refund of the $2,550 I had paid, when Silvia instructed us to close our eyes. Speaking in a low, hypnotic voice, she asked us to slow down our breathing and relax every part of our bodies. After a few minutes of stillness, she directed us to jog our memory until a moment of childhood trauma popped into our minds.

Nothing.

I blinked an eye open to see if there were other skeptics in the room. Everyone else seemed to be in a trance. As hokey as I found the whole thing, I figured I had nothing to lose by playing along. While I began trying to come up with a fake memory to share, a real one surfaced.

I was about four. My father, a maniacal driver, lost control of his car on a narrow mountain road during a family vacation. He had to choose between flying off a cliff or smashing into a truck. He chose the latter, thrusting my older sister and me, who were unrestrained in the back seat, toward the windshield. I had been holding a toy train set, which broke as the car became a jumble of twisted slabs of steel and shattered glass. Miraculously, no one was seriously hurt, but I wailed uncontrollably and held up my disfigured train.

When Silvia spoke after a few minutes of silence, I realized I had failed to comfort little Ernesto, to somehow avert the accident, to find a way to make things right with all the agency and wherewithal that comes with adulthood. Silvia asked us to share our memories and the actions we had taken. I described mine in detail, surprised by the extent to which I had gotten into the whole thing. I admitted that I had become too immersed in the memory to take corrective action. My inner child had been left crying with a broken toy in his hand.

Silvia asked pointedly what the episode revealed about my parents.

"They were irresponsible," I blurted out, much to my surprise.

"Good!" Silvia said.

My parents had been imperfect and dysfunctional at times. But *irresponsible* is not an adjective I previously would have applied to them, particularly concerning my early years. Had Silvia tricked me with her psychobabble into concluding something that didn't quite ring true? Or had I stumbled into something worth examining? I sat uncomfortably as others in the room shared their childhood memories. Silvia interjected with questions that felt like darts, operating like a prosecutor cross-examining an oblivious witness to a conclusion that had become apparent to everyone else in the room except the speaker.

The sun had just set when the session ended. We were encouraged to nap for a bit before making our way in the dark at 10:00 p.m. to the ceremony room up the hill for our first taste of the medicine.

〜〜〜 Some fifteen cots were arranged in a circle in the maloca, the circular ceremony room with a cone-shaped ceiling. Each was outfitted with a pillow, a neatly folded blanket, and a bucket to vomit into. As we picked our spots in the room, trading nervous glances, Silvia and Rohan whispered as they poured ayahuasca into shot glasses. They rely on intuition in deciding how big of a dose will be right for each person, a process that often leads to bargaining and pleas for a more generous pour. I was relieved to get a light dose that first night. When Silvia handed me the glass, I brought it up to my nose. The smell of the thick, dark brown sludge was revolting.

Silvia had us stand in a circle for a quick guided meditation to set an intention for the ceremony.

"Imagine roots shooting down from your feet to the center of the earth," Silvia said. The roots needed to be long and thick to keep us grounded.

I was done playing Silvia's game, so I rolled my eyes discreetly and made no effort to sprout imaginary roots. Each participant had to share an intention.

Princess began by referring to the medicine as "Mother Ayahuasca."

For fuck's sake, I thought.

She was far from alone. Virtually everyone else who had been down this path personified ayahuasca as a wise elder feminine force that was about to enter our bodies like a sacrament.

When it came time to share my intention, I said I wanted to understand what had brought me here. It was simple and felt genuine enough. When the last participant spoke, Silvia asked us to head back to our cots and raise our glasses.

"Have a good journey," she said as the lights were dimmed.

I drank my serving in one gulp. The taste was acrid. My eyes watered as I fought the urge to puke. Silvia began playing gentle music that seemed to be in sync with the sounds of the jungle that poured in through the mesh enveloping the maloca. Frogs croaked. Birds chirped. Insects wailed. Maybe I was imagining it, but there seemed to be a rhythm to the cacophony of jungle sounds. After a while, the wild symphony sounded like the planet's beating heart.

Conjuring that image reminded me of my own medicine-deprived heart. I placed one hand on it and felt its beat quicken. Silvia's music changed abruptly, and suddenly, the room was filled with the pounding of drums. I began worrying that my nervous system was being dangerously revved up and wondered what a stroke would feel like. Would I even notice it coming on amid all the noise?

Then the colors appeared, instantly blasting away the heaviness of fear and the tyranny of thoughts. They were faint streaks of pink and blue at first, unfolding like symmetrical figures in a kaleidoscope. The colors became brighter, the outlines sharper, and the shapes more ornate with every passing moment. I felt paralyzed, surrendering to the majesty of these mysterious visions. Were they a product of my mind? Gifts from another realm? Evidence that Princess was onto something? Or was this simply what it felt like to be on drugs?

I noticed I was smiling as I pondered these questions. Then I felt the unexpected flow of tears that drifted onto the pillow from the corner of my eyes. It didn't feel like conventional crying. There was no heavy breathing, no tightness in my chest, and not a hint of sadness. I had never felt lighter, less burdened. For a few precious moments, the fog of depression cleared, its shackles suddenly unclasped.

The colors receded after what may have been four minutes or an hour. Time is shapeless and squirrelly when you're in the custody of ayahuasca. I yearned for a booster dose, hoping it would yield a second act or at least an encore. As I tried unsuccessfully to bring the light streaks back, my attention shifted abruptly.

Suddenly, I felt the presence of a friend I hadn't seen in years, someone I had thought about only sporadically in the three years since he blew his brains out inside a red pickup truck in Colorado. It felt dreamlike, but absolutely real, hearing Dominic's devilish laugh and seeing his piercing brown eyes. No words were exchanged, but for a few moments, I sensed that a portal had somehow opened and he had dropped in to sit by my side.

Dominic is the closest friend I have lost to suicide. We met in 2008 in Baghdad, where we were among the few openly gay journalists in a tribe of hard-drinking, hard-partying international correspondents. Like me, he shifted to Afghanistan around 2010, when the conflict there surged as the Iraq story became stale.

His final overseas posting was in Pakistan. He was among the first reporters to make it to the safe house where Osama bin Laden was killed in Abbottabad. Dominic smuggled out a brick from the site, which he donated to the September 11 museum in lower Manhattan.

Dominic had always struck me as a man gliding through life, always bursting with the best gossip and regaling me with tales of sexual conquests on far-flung military bases. His violent death in 2014 came as a shock to most of his friends. In a letter explaining his final act, Dominic wrote that he had been experiencing cognitive decline, which he believed had been caused by a concussion from a mortar attack in northern Iraq in 2009 and a bullet that struck his helmet in Afghanistan two years later.

"I cannot live like that," he wrote. "Nor can I bear the thought of those around me watching me degenerate."

I was a few months into my new job at the *Times* when Dominic decided to check out early from life. I wrote a short tribute in the newspaper and grieved his loss for a few days, wishing I had done more to stay in touch. But his memory had faded to the back of my mind, one more file in the repository of awful things that we compartmentalize after the initial shock wears off.

It made no sense that my attention was now entirely focused on Dominic, not merely as a memory but as a presence so real I could almost feel his breath. He seemed at peace. I was briefly tempted to ask questions about his death, as though it were possible to reconfigure the past. Using thoughts, not words, I conveyed to Dominic that I missed him, that I respected his decision, and that I loved seeing him so radiant. The strength of our bond made me feel warm, like a tight embrace.

"Two hours!" Silvia suddenly said as she took tiny steps around the room, observing her participants, little shadows whirling on our cots. "Two hours," she repeated again and again, noting we had reached the point in the ceremony where people could ask for a second dose. Her voice broke the spell of being in the presence of Dominic, who suddenly was nowhere to be found. I heard someone vomit violently into a bucket, making a guttural, gurgling sound.

My stomach was making loud noises, which made the prospect of a second shot unpalatable. This had been plenty for my initiation with the medicine. I listened to the bursts of sounds from the jungle, fell into a thoughtless, trancelike state, and let my tired body drift into a deep sleep.

〰〰 Dawn was a most unwelcome sight when I blinked my eyes open in the ceremony room. There was grainy ayahuasca residue in my mouth. The smell of vomit and the loud snoring of a person I didn't recognize made me want to dart out. I walked unsteadily back to the bungalow, where I lay awake for a couple of hours, feeling that the room was spinning, and waited for breakfast.

I felt silly remembering how real the presence of Dominic had felt the night before. Princess and Silvia had made me impressionable with their starry-eyed tales of the medicine. I had walked right into their trap. Relieved my rational mind was reasserting itself, I vowed to spend the rest of the retreat watching this whole spectacle unfold with detachment, unwilling to become a supporting actor again.

That resolve hardened later in the day when we gathered in the main meeting room, bleary-eyed and still a bit buzzed, for the first "sharing" ceremony. Lucas, the German, said he had realized during the ceremony that he was God, that we're all God, that we're bundles of skin and bones containing bits of divinity. The British therapist spoke in detail about her past life as a Guatemalan amputee. Someone spoke of being visited by aliens who were friendly and intelligent.

There were tearful accounts of newly unearthed memories of sexual abuse and wrenching stories of cruel parents. It felt like watching a reality show in real life.

Listening to the veteran psychonauts, I felt mainly contempt and a sense of superiority. But part of me was envious. There was a refreshing levity in the nuttier folks in the room, a sense that they had transcended the mild neurosis that has become the baseline mood for so many people slogging from one day to the next. Their sparkle made me feel heavy, tense, and insufferably cynical.

I brought that rigidity to the second ceremony, which was a total bust. A heavier dose of the medicine made my thinking foggy and sent me to the toilet with diarrhea. There were no childhood memories, no profound insights, and certainly no psychedelic fireworks this time. I wiggled uncomfortably on my mat, feeling nauseated and fading in and out of consciousness. Sporadic sounds of violent vomiting jolted me to attention every few minutes, and I scanned the shadows in front of me trying to decipher the source of each purge.

I woke up the next morning with nothing to show for another restless night spent on that thin cot. I felt defeated, defrauded, and just plain dumb for putting my body through this torturous experience when I could have taken a relaxing vacation on the beach.

The following day, in preparation for the third ceremony, Silvia put on her "soul retrieval" workshop. Every traumatic or hurtful thing that happens in our lives, she explained, causes a tiny part of our soul to fracture. Over time, souls become like puzzles that begin life complete and perfect and are gradually rendered unrecognizable as one piece after another goes missing. To make matters worse, Silvia said, each hole creates an opportunity for malign "entities" to find a home in our souls and grow like mold.

As luck would have it, Silvia had come up with a method to dislodge entities that didn't serve us. It required scanning our bodies with eyes closed until we stumbled into an intrusive entity. Say you discovered a thorn-shaped entity in your left lung. Silvia instructed us to imagine it being pulled out of our bodies by a powerful cosmic vacuum cleaner that swooped in from the sky. Once the entity was gone, we had to imagine a green laser beam filling the holes in our souls, until they were patched up and good as new.

The vacuum cleaner would be working hard that night in the ceremony room, Silvia said, performing spiritual surgeries all night, doing the painstaking work of patching up busted souls. "The entities are taken to a hospital in another dimension for healing," Silvia explained.

Of course they were.

〰 That night, Silvia and Rohan, who probably had sensed my disappointment, decided I was ready for an even larger dose. I acquiesced, more out of resignation than enthusiasm. After completing the roots meditation and setting our intentions, I gulped down the thick brew in my cup. The gentle music came on, blending placidly with the songs of the wild outside. A soft rain gave the night a cleansing touch.

I found myself yearning again for the light streaks I had seen on the first night, assuming they were the gateway to a good trip. But the medicine had other plans.

About an hour into the ceremony, I felt a sinking feeling, like a stone drifting into a deep pond. My body felt possessed. For the first time, I understood clearly why people refer to this thing as Mother Ayahuasca. I was being led, gently but firmly, by a mysterious feminine force. My autonomy of thought had been hijacked, and somehow it didn't terrify me.

Once I hit bottom, there was a tunnellike structure. As I moved forward involuntarily, I began seeing frames from the past displayed at a dizzying speed. Some were snapshots that vanished the moment I registered them. Others played out like short video clips: A dead charred baby lying on a tray. Western Baghdad. Suicide bombing. The smell of burned hair. *Next.* There's a man holding a gun to my father's head in our living room. That home invasion drags on for hours. One of the gunmen makes a snide remark about a framed photo of me in Disney World. *Next.* I'm sitting on a train to Amsterdam when I tell my older sister I'm gay. I'm nineteen. I'm wearing orange pants. The look of horror on her face. The unbearable silence that follows. *Next.* I walk in on my father masturbating. He trips as he lurches out of bed to turn off porn playing from a VCR. My first glimpse of intercourse.

I was dazzled by the vividness of these memories. I recognized each as being a faithful rendering of a snippet of the past. What was particularly mesmerizing was that I retrieved not only the information but also the feeling each moment had evoked, as though I were rewinding the tape, then speeding way ahead, reliving random parts of the past with dreamlike precision.

Suddenly, the blast of disparate moments stopped, and I was plunged into the arms of a man whose name I hadn't uttered in years. Diego. We're on his sofa, my head resting on his chest. His teeth are yellow. There are two glasses of red wine on the table in front of us. There always were. His bushy beard has streaks of gray. He caresses my arm. I notice the liver spots on his hand.

This was my first taste of falling in love with a man. I was eighteen. He was fifty-two. He was funny and wily, well versed in seduction. I was starved for parental love. I was drawn into the memory of us with ravenous curiosity, hooked on a loop of moments we shared. I didn't get a linear narrative, only fragments that bounced back and forth in time:

One day he shows up with a gift, a hardcover edition of T. S. Eliot's *Old Possum's Book of Practical Cats*. Next.

We're on a sailing boat and he calls me the most beautiful man who ever lived. I'm so happy I hope the boat never finds its way to shore. *Next.* At a restaurant, when I order cheesecake, he remarks I've put on weight. *Next.*

We're checking into a hotel in northern Florida. He asks me to wait outside. He doesn't want the attendant in the lobby to see the two bodies that will share the king-size bed in the room. *Next.* When it all unravels, when we're the talk of the town, I sit across from him in his living room and watch him sob.

"It was never going to last," he says. He hands me a final gift, a poem he wrote comparing his heart to an old Cadillac in Havana, barreling down a hill with flimsy brakes.

〰 I woke up the next morning drowning in grief. I thought of Silvia's inner child workshop and desperately wanted to turn back time to edit out that destabilizing relationship. At the very least, I yearned to give the heartbroken teenager I saw overnight a hug, to tell him things would turn out just fine.

My skepticism about the power of ayahuasca was blasted away. Back in my room, I furiously took notes about the retrieved memories, fearing they might slip back into the darker corners of my mind.

I realized I had no idea if Diego was still alive. He would be in his early seventies. I couldn't decide whether falling into his orbit did more harm than good or whether he did more to mend or break my heart. Suddenly, Silvia's metaphor of tattered souls made perfect sense. This relationship left a gaping hole in mine, opening the door for feelings of indignity and regret that had metastasized over the years. I was carrying them around like bricks in a backpack, a self-imposed punishment for a perceived sin I was not done atoning for.

I sat on the terrace of the bungalow absorbing this painful insight while playing a country cover of "Amazing Grace" on repeat. With tears flowing, I saw the relationship in a broader context: as a driving force for a series of decisions that shaped my adult life. I remembered the awful letter my mother wrote after word of my relationship with Diego got around, in which she used the word *maricón*, faggot. My father was less outwardly judgmental, but I recall the sadness in his eyes. I caught wind of how classmates in Colombia had reacted. I dreaded ever seeing the girl I dated in high school again.

It saddened me to realize how many of my decisions had been driven by an unconscious quest to atone. It made perfect sense why I had been so reluctant to attend family weddings and funerals over the years, always feeling on some level like a pariah. I realized that my professional success, to a large extent, had been built on a foundation of shame and a desperate desire never to have to return home.

When I shared some of these thoughts later in the day with the group, I was a sobbing mess. I'd inserted myself back into the spectacle, this time wholeheartedly. I told Silvia she was right in sensing I was repressing something. She nodded warmly. Princess looked at me with compassion, and I felt sorry for all the mean thoughts that had crossed my mind about her throughout the week.

When I stopped speaking and my tears stopped flowing, I noticed something startling. My heartbeat was imperceptible. My blood pressure had slowed. Something had shifted within me. A couple of days before the retreat was to end, there was no question in my mind: If this was actually a cult, I definitely wanted in.

〰 The day we left, Rohan posted a quote on a whiteboard used for daily schedule updates. "Nothing changes, just the view," it read. But in fact, this experience had fundamentally jolted my mind and lifted my mood. Loops of obsessive, dark thoughts, so often the grist of depression, had given way to a more expansive and curious perception of the present moment. I knew virtually nothing then about the neuroscience of depression or the emerging theories about how psychedelics alter brain function and mood. But in the immediate aftermath, I experienced a sublime sense of calm, which made evident the extent to which anxiety and a constant sense of foreboding had become my default setting.

Recent advances in neuroimaging have given scientists a glimpse into how depression plays out in the brain. People who have attempted suicide experience a decrease of gray matter in key areas of the brain responsible for regulating emotional responses and impulse control, according to a 2017 study by researchers at Yale University. Brain scans of suicidal people have also showed decreased blood flow among regions of the brain, which indicates a degradation in neural links. That has led researchers to conclude that depression can be a symptom of an atrophying brain, which gradually loses the ability to reason, keep perspective, and regulate emotions.

Taking psychedelics like ayahuasca appears to have the opposite effect. These compounds seem to enhance the brain's wiring system, enabling richer interaction among neural networks. "Brain activity becomes less predictable, faster, more random, more entropic," said Dr. Robin Carhart-Harris, a professor of neurology and psychiatry at the University of California, San Francisco, who has done pioneering research on psychedelics using brain scans. During a trip, this phenomenon often creates a dizzying array of visions, thoughts, and perceptions. When the mental dust settles, often people are left with profound insights about the nature of their suffering and gain an ability to make valuable associations and inferences about their past. Neurologists refer to this as a period of enhanced neuroplasticity, a reference to the brain's ability to make new and stronger connections.

With support from a skilled therapist, this state of disruptive thinking and perception can be extraordinarily clarifying and therapeutic, setting in motion long-lasting, and at times permanent, changes in outlook and behavior, Robin told me.

This emerging field of medicine has deep and complex roots. For starters, it's important to acknowledge that Indigenous people have been using psychoactive plants for centuries in spiritual and healing rituals. Their use of compounds like ayahuasca, mescaline, and psilocybin far predates the term *psychedelic*, which was coined in the 1950s by the British psychiatrist Humphry Osmond. He was among a group of researchers who became convinced that mind-altering substances like LSD, a synthetic hallucinogen discovered in the 1940s, could revolutionize the treatment of mental illness and addiction.

At a gathering of the New York Academy of Sciences in 1957, Osmond proposed a new word for this class of drugs that profoundly altered cognition and perception. Psychedelic—which blended two Greek words—*psychē* and *dēlein*, or "mind manifesting"—aptly captured the wondrous ability of these compounds to reveal essential elements of ourselves, he argued.

But the nascent field soon fell into disrepute, largely as a result of the work of two Harvard University psychology professors who became psychedelic evangelists. In the early 1960s, the scholars Timothy Leary and Richard Alpert led a series of wild experiments with psychedelics that became known as the Harvard Psilocybin Project. High on hype and short on rigor, the studies turbocharged the appeal of psychedelics on college campuses, injecting a volatile element to the counterculture movement convulsing the nation during the Vietnam era.

As more young people took psychedelics in unstructured settings, many had discombobulating trips. That fueled a wave of alarming press reports about drugs like LSD, which were said to turn sane people psychotic and deranged. Soon came a withering backlash.

In June 1971, President Richard Nixon addressed the nation to declare that drug abuse had become "public enemy number one." Fighting it, the president said, required waging a global "all-out offensive."

The previous year, the United States Congress had passed the Controlled Substances Act, which remains the backbone of drug prohibition. Most countries soon fell in line. The war on drugs set in motion an era of mass incarceration and fueled a flurry of armed conflicts across the globe. As a consequence, it became all but impossible to continue researching the therapeutic potential of psychedelics.

By the 1980s, the few therapists who continued to treat patients with psychedelics worked in the underground. Only a handful of them remained outspoken enthusiasts of the drugs. Key among them was the Czech psychiatrist Stanislav Grof, whose 1980 book on the history of LSD psychotherapy argued that prohibition had senselessly shortchanged psychiatry.

"Psychedelics, used responsibly and with proper caution, would be for psychiatry what the microscope is for biology or the telescope is for astronomy," Grof wrote. "These tools make it possible to study important processes that under normal circumstances are not available for direct observation."

〰 Returning home from the retreat, I was astonished by how profoundly the experience had changed me. It felt as though my emotional hard drive had been restored to factory settings and my senses had been recalibrated. Classical music elicited utter joy, which I had not felt in a long time. I began spending more time in nature, suddenly captivated by the otherworldly hue of the yellow and purple orchids that grow on the bark of old trees in my neighborhood. I stood with reverence in front of a stately *Ceiba pentandra*, observing how its fingerlike roots dug into the earth and ripped open sidewalks with a subtle but unmistakable sense of agency.

To my astonishment—and that of close friends—I completely lost my appetite for alcohol after returning from Spirit Vine and remained a teetotaler since. The first time I ordered steak after the recommended post-retreat diet restrictions had lifted, I found myself cutting into the meat with disgust. It dawned on me that I was chewing on tiny slabs of a dismembered animal, its blood sloshing on my plate. In the weeks that followed, I also gave up eating chicken and fish and became vegetarian. A diet I had long associated with self-righteous anemics made me feel stronger and lighter than ever before. During our retreat, Silvia had spoken effusively about the benefits of a plant-based diet. In my post-retreat afterglow, that message resonated deeply, upending habits and cravings that had shaped my eating choices since childhood.

I began meditating each morning, a ritual that became a means to continue to plumb the dark corners of the mind in a more sustainable manner. My blood pressure fell to a healthy range without drugs. After a few months, elated, I flushed the pills that remained in my quinapril bottle down the toilet. My appetite for no-strings-attached sex abated as I became more mindful that those encounters often left me feeling enervated and alone. My suicidal ideation vanished, suddenly seeming like a nightmare from which I'd awakened. I was dumbfounded by the sum of these changes, in large part because they snapped into place so effortlessly and intuitively. It was as though my mind had been reengineered by a wise external force.

Over the next few years, I spent roughly half of my vacation time going on ayahuasca retreats, paying visits to Silvia and a couple of her competitors for tune-ups. I did this in part because I continued to feel the gravitational pull of depression, which had become a subtler and more manageable force in my life, but by no means a vanquished monster. My guiding theory was that continuing down this path might give me the upper hand. Partaking in dozens of ceremonies brought to the surface a torrent of meaningful memories of childhood, of homeland, of lovers past, and of traumatic events I covered as a journalist.

Each trip seemed to add clarity to my personal narrative, like a puzzle that gradually starts resembling a landscape as pieces snap together. It was painstaking and often grueling work that filled me with wonder about the nature of the mind, of consciousness, and of the healing process. The implicit deal you make on this path is to periodically set aside time and energy to lean heavily into your darkness in order to morph pain and trauma that have been repressed.

I was mightily tempted to join the ranks of the true believers—to double down on a quest to overcome the curse of depression that has been in my bloodline for generations. The power of these psychoactive plants to alter lives and realign priorities was breathtaking. I met former ruthless corporate types who became spiritual seekers overnight, growing out bushy beards and adopting morning breath work and chanting routines. I spoke to people who had walked away from careers and marriages unblinkingly after getting "downloads" from the plants. Some became messianic in their devotion to ayahuasca, self-appointed foot soldiers of a plant realm they think is pulling humans into its orbit before we become sicker and more destructive as a species.

But it didn't take long for my journalistic training to kick in as red flags emerged. Among the innovative and thoughtful healers within this nascent unregulated marketplace for alternative mental health care, I found plenty of scammers, predators, and charlatans. I spoke to women who had been abused by supposed healers. I heard from people who experienced psychotic breakdowns and paranoid delusions after tripping. I met retreat participants persuaded to spend money in reckless ways.

It bothered me that as retreats grew more sophisticated and expensive, the role of Indigenous people became increasingly marginal, at times blatantly ornamental.

I wanted to understand what led to the transformation I experienced after my first brush with ayahuasca and the extent to which it was replicable for other people struggling with depression. So I decided to spend most of the next year documenting how this Wild West of medicinal psychedelics came to be and how it's changing the way we think about mental health and drug use.

This journey began taking shape as I was mourning the death of my father, Jamie Londoño, who died in the fall of 2020 from an aggressive cancer. Losing my father rekindled a curiosity that was sparked during my first retreat at Spirit Vine. I had long known that mental illness had deep roots in my family tree. But it was only after we buried him that I began piecing together a painful history that made my own struggles make a lot more sense.

3 A LINEAGE OF UNSTABLE MINDS

SHORTLY BEFORE MY FATHER DIED, he recounted an old story that had always struck me as odd. In January 1977, as the day of his wedding to my mother approached, well after the church was booked and the invitations were mailed out, my father said he asked her to see a psychiatrist. One session was all he asked for, a perfunctory screening he hoped would give him the all clear to bind their fates. It was the spousal equivalent of a home inspection, and to me, it signaled that he walked down the aisle with a premonition, a nagging fear that he might be marrying an unsound woman.

The day after he died, sorting through the drawers in his bedroom, I found a thick stack of antidepressant prescriptions amid tattered letters, newspaper clippings, and yellowing utility bills. I knew my father had often been sad and lonely in his final years, as his already small social circle dwindled, his memory became blurry, and minor setbacks and annoyances morphed in his mind into catastrophic problems. But as I leafed through the prescriptions, which spanned years and several psychiatrists, it struck me that our conversations about depression had been guarded. We hinted at times about the ways in which we were struggling, but we were reluctant to linger on the subject too long, to discuss it frankly, perhaps fearing that speaking openly about depression would breathe life into it, making it more intractable.

My grief over his death was imbued with regret over the conversations that could have been and set in motion a quest to piece together the recent history of distress in my family tree. Depression often feels like a personal failing, so documenting that I was part of a long lineage of unstable minds prone to despondency, extreme melancholy, and distorted thinking offered a glimmer of absolution. I came to see it as part of my heritage. This raised an intriguing question: Is it possible to short-circuit a generational wave of suffering, to somehow transmute the sorrow and despair that has been lurking in our DNA for generations? And might the kind of mind-bending, body-jolting trips I had been drawn to, time and again, be a means to that kind of cleansing? To answer those questions, I first had to learn a bit about heredity.

〰〰 Scientists have long suspected that some people are genetically more prone to depression. Until relatively recently, they relied largely on studies involving twins raised separately to test that theory. Those studies were limited by small sample sizes and other variables that made it difficult to draw firm conclusions. In recent years, however, scientific breakthroughs in deciphering the human genetic code and connecting it to our traits have left little doubt that our genes shape a person's risk for depression. Drawing on massive datasets of human DNA samples, scientists have found that many individuals who have been diagnosed with major depressive disorder share a number of common genetic variants.

"We're at a really exciting time in the field of psychiatric genetics," Dr. Erin C. Dunn, a psychiatric epidemiologist at Harvard University, told me. "What we are learning is that there are hundreds, if not thousands, of variants that relate to our risk" for depression.

Beyond the set of genetic variants we're born with, researchers have also begun to study the role that epigenetics plays in mental illness. This field, in which Dr. Dunn is an expert, considers how a person's environment and behavior—and even those of their parents and grandparents—affect the expression of their genes. While the sequence of genes we are born with is largely immutable, scientists have come to believe that our environment and experiences alter the expression of our genes in ways that can ripple across generations. They have documented this by studying the descendants of people who endured famines and the children of Holocaust survivors. The latter were found to have a high incidence of depression and anxiety.

I asked Dr. Dunn if she thought psychedelics have the potential to unburden us from ancestral trauma. She said the prospect was plausible given that hallucinogenic trips have been shown to enhance neuroplasticity. "It's not impossible to imagine that using psychedelics helps to induce the brain to be in a more plastic state that then allows for new neural connections to be made and, potentially, for unhelpful connections to be weakened," she said.

But for now, there's a simple and applicable takeaway from what we've learned about genetics and mental health, Dr. Dunn said. Many families, including her own, have done a lousy job of speaking candidly about mental health challenges. Dr. Dunn told me she only learned as an adult that one of her uncles had died by suicide. Years later, when her grandmother passed away, Dr. Dunn learned there was more to the story. In a box of mementos her grandmother kept was a newspaper clipping describing how her uncle, as a child, had discovered the body of his mother, who also took her own life.

"My mother never wanted to talk about it or confront these painful realities, because for her it was easier to just keep them in the past," Dr. Dunn said. "But starting to ask questions within your family to better understand where you come from and what might lie ahead could be helpful."

This is what I would set out to do.

〰 When I was growing up, I knew that my maternal grandfather, Hernando Martínez, had an epic unraveling and that he died at a psychiatric hospital in Bogotá, where he had languished for years. I also had heard that my paternal grandmother, Natalia Jaramillo, had become a zealous believer in Freudian psychoanalysis, but I knew little about what sparked her interest.

When I began calling relatives who had been close to both grand-parents, who'd died more than forty years ago, I was surprised by how eager they were to talk.

Before I started making calls to ask about Hernando's life, this is what I knew: He had been a doting father of eight and had been devoted to my grandmother Carlota. He had been among the most successful and prolific civil engineers of his generation, at times tak-ing on more projects than he could reasonably handle. In his late fifties, he unraveled as bouts of mania followed by periods of depres-sion, once manageable, intensified. By the time he died of a stroke in August 1981, he had been committed to a psychiatric hospital for nearly a decade. My mother, Margarita Martínez, spoke about him infrequently during my childhood, and I never asked her about his life. It was a long-overdue conversation.

Hernando was born in October 1917 in Bogotá, the capital, to par-ents from Popayán, a city in southwestern Colombia wedged between two mountain ranges. The youngest of twelve children, he grew up in a family scarred by grief. He received the name of a brother who died as a toddler before Hernando was born, as though his birth repre-sented a second coming. Years later, his sister Elisa, who helped raise him, died at sixteen. He had an extraordinary talent for math, my uncle Eduardo, Hernando's oldest son, told me. "He was fascinated by numbers and could make complicated calculations in his mind," Eduardo said. Soon after graduating from the National University of Colombia in Bogotá, he joined the construction firm led by his brother Ignacio, who had a knack for winning major government contracts. Hernando loved being in the field, and he took the lead managing day-to-day operations at construction sites. But managing Hernando was no easy task. From an early age, he exhibited dra-matic mood swings that led a small cluster of relatives to spring into action to contain him and keep him out of sight when he was unwell, Eduardo told me. At the time, *depression* was not a widely used term, and there was a dearth of effective treatment options. At the urging of relatives, Hernando was treated with insulin shock therapy, an intervention that induced a state of coma, and with electroshock therapy. "This was handled with utmost secrecy because it was understood that a person who had a mental disorder was very unlikely to get married," Eduardo said.

The coverup worked. In his early thirties, Hernando married my grandmother, Carlota Zuleta, who came from a prominent political family. My grandmother, who was only nineteen, soon realized there was something amiss with the man she had promised to stick with in sickness and in health. Soon after getting married, my grandmother got pregnant with their first child, Himelda, and Hernando plunged into the first of several depressive episodes of his married life.

After weeks of moping around the house, bleary-eyed and weepy, he would boomerang into phases of ebullience, leaning into business opportunities with boundless optimism and showering my grandmother with affection. He would act impulsively when he was feeling great. One day, for instance, he came home and announced that he had fallen in love with a country house in La Unión, a town a few hours from the capital, and decided to buy it on a whim. If my grandmother was alarmed by her husband's mood swings during the early years of their marriage, she didn't show it. She comforted him during low points and celebrated his periods of mania, backing him resolutely when he took on dubious business ventures. "He would get depressed at times, but it was mild," Eduardo told me. "My mom was aware of it, my dad was aware of it, but life went on."

Hernando's manic states were often good for business. His firm won a contract to build two major projects in the capital: the military hospital and the new headquarters of the Bank of Colombia, a twenty-story building that would be, at the time, the tallest in the city. He gravitated toward high-risk, high-reward ventures, including one in a city roiled by violence, to which he seemed impervious. "He had an infinite capacity for work. He would work twenty hours a day," Eduardo said. He won contracts to build housing units for university students and purchased a big lot to build a working-class residential complex. Outside of work, he relished taking his older children on long hikes, horseback rides, and waterskiing excursions. "He taught us to love reading, he taught us to love sports," my mother told me. "It was a magical childhood."

Eduardo told me that the first time his father's behavior rattled him came when he was in third grade, attending a school that his parents helped found. One morning, as Eduardo was getting ready for class, Hernando told him not to bother, that he was never going to set foot in that school again. The reason was perplexing. The night before, Hernando explained, there had been a showdown during a school board meeting over a psychologist who had been hired to counsel students. Perhaps resenting the experimental treatments he had been subjected to earlier in life, Hernando had a deep distrust of anything that sounded like psychiatry, Eduardo said. So after a majority of board members voted to keep the psychologist, he withdrew Eduardo and one of his brothers. "It was impulsive, imposing his views on the friends with whom he had founded the school," Eduardo said. "He effectively said: 'If you don't do what I say, my children are out.'"

Around that time, in 1962, Hernando's brother Ignacio died, depriving him of the relative who had fostered his immense talents and reined in his most self-destructive impulses.

The death and the fight over the psychologist led to another hasty decision: Hernando and Carlota withdrew their other children from school and within days bought one-way plane tickets to the United States.

"The whole family boarded a plane and, not speaking any English, arrived in New York," Eduardo said. Hernando rented a large furnished house in Greenwich, Connecticut, and an expensive office in Wall Street, intending to break into the construction business in the

United States. But he never made a dime in the United States, and providing for eight children made their savings evaporate, Eduardo recalled.

That's when Hernando sank into the first major depressive episode that shook the whole family. "He would chew on a handkerchief and pace back and forth with a withdrawn gaze," Eduardo told me. Himelda, the eldest daughter, who was eleven at the time, remembers her father would languish in bed for days on end, not bothering to shave.

After a little over a year abroad, after Hernando failed to find work, the family returned to Bogotá in August 1962. Hernando continued to unravel rapidly and dramatically. Having squandered the family savings in the United States, he dashed off to neighboring Venezuela, booked a room at a fancy hotel, and threw a party for bankers and other power brokers in the oil-rich nation, hoping to walk away with fresh construction deals. None materialized. He was so cash-strapped by then that a relative had to wire money to settle the hotel bill, Eduardo recalled. "He returned home severely depressed," Eduardo said. After bouncing back, he made a similar trip to a couple of cities in Colombia that only added to the family's debt. By then, his behavior was so outlandish that relatives took him to a psychiatric ward for the first of several interventions. "He went totally bankrupt and became depressed," Eduardo said.

When my grandmother saw fit to take control of the family finances in 1967, she realized her husband had used their home as collateral for a loan and that they were about to get evicted. She hospitalized him, Eduardo said. In the years that followed, Carlota became the sole breadwinner, working initially as a principal at an all-girls Catholic school. For a while, Hernando bounced back and forth between the family's new rented home and psychiatric wards as Carlota toggled between despair and compassion. "When he was severely depressed or severely manic, she would take him to the hospital," Eduardo said, and the family would get an out-of-sight, out-of-mind reprieve for a month or two. "Then she would go visit him, and regardless of how he was doing, she would bring him back home because she couldn't bear seeing him in that state."

Carlota refused to speak about Hernando's frequent hospitalizations with her children, and they developed no vocabulary to make sense of what their father had become. But one day, in his late teens, Eduardo showed up unannounced at the office of Dr. Alfonso Uribe, a physician who was a friend of the family. When he was ushered into the office, Eduardo cut to the chase. "Dr. Uribe, I want to know what is wrong with my father," he remembered saying. Two giant tears streamed down the doctor's cheeks. "He was very moved, and it took him a while to gather his thoughts," Eduardo recalled.

"That was the question I was afraid you might ask," Dr. Uribe finally said. "It's also the question I hoped you would ask."

Dr. Uribe pulled a thick book titled *Family Encyclopedia of Medicine and Health* from a bookshelf, opened it to page 631, and pointed to a subhead that read: "Manic Depressive Psychosis." The book said the condition was as common as schizophrenia and that it affected nearly a third of patients committed to psychiatric wards. "It is characterized by periodic cycles of mania and depression," Eduardo read. "During the manic phase, the person can display tremendous energy, incessant activity and exaggerated wellbeing." Patients reported the high points of their mood swings as pleasurable and often displayed delusions of grandeur and an effervescent libido, according to the book. But the flip side was crushing, the book warned. Patients become "dangerously depressed and miserable . . . and sink into a state of deep despair over a feeling that they are to blame for sins and mistakes that are often illusory." People with manic depression often become suicidal, "deeming themselves unworthy of being alive," the book said. The last paragraph of the section didn't provide much reason for hope: "Complete recoveries are rare."

Dr. Uribe told Eduardo that Hernando was a textbook case of the condition and that he was aware of a number of other cases in the

Martínez family. Dr. Uribe said there were new drugs that were being used to stabilize psychiatric patients, but cautioned that they often did more harm than good. Freudian psychoanalysis was an option, but unlikely to tame a mind prone to spiraling up and down. Finally, Dr. Uribe said, there was an extreme measure he would strenuously advise against. Some doctors had begun performing partial lobotomies on manic-depressive patients, he said, removing a slice of the brain that regulates "affection." In the best of cases, Dr. Uribe said, "you're left with a person who can think and move, but who is devoid of feelings."

〰〰 With a diagnosis in hand, Eduardo persuaded Hernando to meet with a pair of doctors. Hernando bristled at the suggestion that his mind was malfunctioning. When one doctor suggested trying experimental drugs, Hernando shut him down and began rambling about his plan to turn the family's fortunes around. He wanted to start a business importing Cadillacs. Everyone in the family told him the idea was doomed; he had no capital to get it started and lacked experience in the field. Hernando was crushed.

"You've lost faith in me," he told Eduardo, visibly hurt. Soon, Hernando's dejection morphed into anger. One day, he assaulted Eduardo. The family called a doctor, and soon a team of nurses from the Clínica Montserrat, a psychiatric hospital in Bogotá, arrived at the house armed with a syringe filled with a sedative. "They sedated him and took him away to be hospitalized," Eduardo said. "It was very traumatic to have reached that extreme."

From that point, Hernando left the psychiatric ward on rare occasions. He would put on a suit when his children visited and conveyed more sadness than resentment over his confinement. But visits grew infrequent because seeing him in that state was crushingly sad.

"My mom convinced us that *Papi* suffered enormously every time we went to visit," my mother told me. That much was evident, my mother added, recalling how he would try to plead, barter, and beg to return home. "Get me out of here, I'm desperate," she remembers him saying. "Don't leave me here. I want to escape."

But no one wanted to be responsible for taking care of him outside the hospital, so his pleas went unheeded and visits became ever-more infrequent over the years, my mother said. "He was a good father, supremely sweet," my mother said. "When I close my eyes and think about it, I get profoundly sad."

On special occasions, like weddings and graduations, Hernando got to leave the hospital for a few hours. He would get glimpses of how the skyline he had helped build was getting taller and denser. Standing alongside relatives who had effectively given up on him, he readily flashed a smile posing for photos marking family milestones.

During one of his final outings, Hernando wore a tuxedo to walk my mother down the aisle. I can't help wondering what gossip was exchanged and whether guests held their breath as he dutifully played his ceremonial role. In black-and-white photos published in the social pages of the newspaper, he appears smiling, seemingly grateful to have been allowed into the realm of the sane, even for a few hours.

Eduardo said that in his final years, Hernando's mood stabilized somewhat after he was given lithium, which by then had become a common treatment for bipolar disorder. But there was never serious consideration of bringing him home.

My mother picked up Hernando from the hospital for the last time a few weeks after I was born in late April 1981, so he could meet his first grandson. Hernando sat on a rocking chair in our living room and swayed gently as he held me on his lap, my mother told me. He wore a beige sweater with a V-neck and a dark tie. "This is the most darling baby in the world," my mother recalls him saying. When it was time to leave, Hernando asked her to pick him up from the hospital again soon. "Come back often," he pleaded, a request that somehow did not convey a trace of bitterness. "I want to see you. Please. Don't leave me all alone there."

A few months later, on the morning of August 18, my mother was breastfeeding me in that same rocking chair when the phone rang. Anita, the nanny who helped raise me, barreled into the living room looking panicked. Carlota was on the phone, she said. "It's very, very urgent," Anita said.

Pulling me away from feeding, my mother walked over to the kitchen and picked up the phone.

"Your father just died," Carlota said flatly. "Heart attack."

My mother felt her knees buckle and her body jolt. She handed me over to Anita and for the next few seconds wondered if her body would produce another drop of milk.

"I thought to myself, *My milk is now poisoned*," she told me, relaying the type of irrational concern that becomes paramount in the early stages of grief. "*What will I feed this baby?*"

〰〰 A framed photo of Hernando holding me as a baby in that rocking chair was displayed in the living room of my childhood home alongside one of my paternal grandmother, Natalia. The latter, a black-and-white portrait, shows a gray-haired woman with a withdrawn gaze kneeling in a rose garden. Growing up, I had a vague awareness of Hernando's turbulent life. But no one ever mentioned that mental illness afflicted the other branch of my family tree. Natalia, it turns out, also spent long periods at the Clínica Montserrat undergoing experimental treatments for depression.

I became intensely interested in her life following my father's death. The night before he succumbed to Merkel cell carcinoma, a rare form of skin cancer, he cried out deliriously in bed. The nurse who was tending to him said much of what he said was unintelligible. But at one point, the nurse later told us, my father, who was staunchly agnostic and believed neither in heaven nor hell, lurched his arms skyward. "Natalia!" he exclaimed, time and again, with childlike wonder and pining. "Natalia. Natalia. Natalia." The name meant nothing to the nurse, but when she relayed the scene early the next morning, shortly before my father's heart rattled to a halt, we were at once haunted and relieved. The possibility that Natalia had attended to his agonizing death seemed fitting. After all, they both narrowly escaped death some seventy-eight years back when he was born.

〰〰 Natalia Jaramillo was born in January 1915, in Ibagué, a city in western Colombia in the foothills of a majestic snowcapped volcano. She was the eldest of three daughters born to Hernando Jaramillo and Sara Restrepo. Martín Restrepo, one of her grandfathers, was a cunning businessman who used profits from gold mines and coffee plantations to buy a massive estate called Hacienda Tolima, which was bursting with waterfalls and hot springs.

When the girls were young, Hernando and Sara boarded a trans-oceanic ship and moved the family to London. Natalia and her sisters learned to speak English with native fluency, and within a few years, the family resettled in Paris so the girls could pick up French.

Spooked by the rise of Nazism in Europe, Hernando and Sara returned home in 1934, where they found their fortune suddenly threatened in a profoundly changed nation. *Colonos*, or squatters, were invading estates like Martín Restrepo's. Left-leaning politicians, who were ascendant at the time, took the side of the *colonos* and called for sweeping land reforms designed to distribute wealth and opportunity more equitably. Martín fought vigorously to protect his estate as land conflicts proliferated. A law in 1936 gave squatters— many of them humble peasants—the upper hand in land rights disputes, which set in motion the sudden dissolution of a vast fortune.

Natalia was nineteen when the family returned to Colombia. Just months after her homecoming, she fell in love with Camilo Londoño, my grandfather, a tall man with blue eyes and a devotion to nature. They were strikingly different. She had spent her formative years in Europe, soaking up the culture London and Paris had to offer. Camilo was happiest getting around on horseback and drank bitter-tasting plant juices he called medicinal. Soon after getting married, Natalia and Camilo moved to a parcel within the ever-shrinking family estate, called Pontevedra, where she gave birth to four children in close succession. Pontevedra had breathtaking views of the volcano and several hot springs that Camilo hailed as powerfully healing.

After Martín died in 1937, Sara, Hernando, and their daughters moved to Bogotá, seeking refuge from the rising violence and restlessness that gripped the countryside. Natalia had long been conflicted about raising a family in the countryside, but my father's birth was the final straw, convincing her she had to leave. She developed a serious infection during labor. As she was fading in and out of consciousness, she would later tell relatives, Camilo had her sign over the property deed to his name, which left her penniless. Farmworkers carried Natalia and her newborn on a hammock hoisted on a rod for miles to get to the nearest road and then to a hospital. After recovering, she made the harrowing trek in reverse and announced to Camilo that she was taking the children to the capital. He regarded the announcement as a tantrum that would pass and locked up the horses on the estate to prevent her from leaving. But Natalia was resolute. Borrowing a neighbor's horses, she and the children left the log cabin behind and headed to the city.

Natalia stayed with relatives in Bogotá while the gravity of her decision sank in. Divorce was exceedingly rare at the time and few women were breadwinners, but Natalia turned to her sole marketable skill. "My mother realized that she didn't know how to do anything, but she spoke English," my father's only living sibling, Hernando, who goes by Nando, told me. Natalia got a job as a secretary at the United States embassy in Bogotá and made extra money translating official documents at night. She pawned her jewelry and leaned on the generosity of her sisters, who were better off, to put food on the table and buy clothes for the children. "She worked like crazy and sold everything she had," Nando recalled, and even so, "we were always completely broke."

Nando has two salient memories from their childhood. One was a nightly ritual during which her children would climb onto Natalia's bed as she read from a twenty-volume encyclopedia for children called

The Treasure of Youth. The other is that Natalia would cry, sometimes for hours, virtually every evening after returning from work. The intensity of her sorrow is haunting to consider now, Nando told me recently. "She was a mother who would cry every night, who slept little, who was always anguished, so clearly we had a mother who was ill," he said. "But we didn't know that other mothers weren't like that. We had no frame of reference."

Curious to learn more about the roots of her sadness, I called a cousin of my father's who sent me a warm condolence message after my father's death. The cousin had reached out after reading a tribute I wrote following his passing, in which I made an allusion to our depression.

The cousin said he wanted to share a well-kept secret surrounding the death of Natalia's father, Hernando Jaramillo, who passed away in October 1939, just short of his seventieth birthday. At the time, the family had said he had died of a heart attack, slumped over a desk where he spent hours drawing sketches on a notepad.

But several years later, during a centennial celebration of Hernando's life, the cousin told me his mother let him in on what had been a shameful family secret. Hernando had struggled with depression for much of his life, and his mood darkened as the family fortune vanished suddenly. "I want you to know that your grandfather died under very difficult circumstances," the cousin recalled his mother saying.

As they processed the shock, Hernando's immediate relatives hastily disposed of any evidence of suicide. "In 1939, a suicide was a tragedy because the person could not be buried in a Catholic cemetery," the cousin explained. "So they made a pact of silence."

Natalia's depression grew so severe that she tried electroshock therapy, an experimental treatment at the time, at a small clinic near her home. "They would wire her all over the body and turn on a generator that produced powerful electric shocks," Nando told me. "It was horrible, but I think it left her with a notable sense of calm." The reprieve was short-lived. When her children were teenagers,

Natalia at one point grew so despondent that she checked into the Clínica Montserrat for a few months. The psychiatrist who treated her turned Natalia into an evangelist for Freudian psychoanalysis, which she insisted all her children undergo.

"It was exotic to have an aunt who was in psychoanalysis," the cousin said. When he was entering adolescence, he told me, Natalia sat him down one day to give him a crash course on sexuality. "She opened a window about something my parents never spoke about," he said.

Several months after the cousin told me this story, he asked if I would consider withholding his name. The request struck me as odd all these years later, yet it's in line with a longstanding aversion to speak openly about our struggles.

Natalia's depression subsided as her children left home, launched careers, and began getting married. But there was a melancholic air about her that never abated. Years of sleepless nights and frantic, anxious days made her hair gray and thin and her body brittle. Her blood pressure had always been stubbornly high and her circulation poor. When making ends meet stopped being a daily scramble, the focus of her attention was a rose garden that she tended to with devotion. It gave her solace to watch rosebuds unfurl slowly until they found their most radiant expression under the sun, only to ultimately wither and drift back onto the moist soil.

One morning when she was sixty-three, she told my father, who was alone with her at home, that she was feeling poorly. He asked whether she wanted to go to a hospital, but she declined. "Take me out to see life," she said, an awkwardly phrased request by which she meant she wanted to see her garden. My father obliged and soon walked her back to bed and sat by her side. Moments later, Natalia's body jerked up slightly and she made a yelping sound. She had succumbed to a stroke.

〜〜 In July 2022, I traveled to Barichara, a small colonial town in the mountains of Colombia, to visit Carlota, my maternal grandmother and the sole grandparent I grew up knowing. Shortly after retiring in 2012 from running a travel agency that kept the family financially afloat after her husband's unraveling, she moved to Barichara and built a house next to hers that she called *la casa de Ernesto*—Ernesto's house. The gesture rankled some of my twenty cousins, but Coquis, as we called her, strong-willed and blunt to a fault, said she had every right to have a favorite grandchild. The two-story house, which has a broad terrace overlooking the bucolic town, was meant to entice me to visit often. It was evident that she was lonely and cherished my company. I managed to get to Barichara every year or two but always left with a nagging feeling that my visits had been too infrequent and brief. When I last visited in October 2019, it was clear that Coquis's memory was faltering. She would tell the same anecdote four times in the span of ten minutes and would repeatedly ask questions I had answered seconds earlier.

I had been warned that her cognitive decline had worsened over the last year, so when I walked into her bedroom shortly after sunset on a Sunday evening, I was guardedly optimistic that she would remember me. But as I walked toward the lounge chair where she was watching a ballet on television, she met me with an icy glare. I knelt down and tentatively reached for her hand. She pulled back and took quick, agitated breaths. I explained who I was, but that did nothing to ease her distress and hostility.

I left her alone that night and lay awake until dawn, feeling shaken by our encounter. I had hoped that during the week ahead I might find a small treasure or two within her vanishing memory. I was especially eager to ask about Hernando, wondering if there was anything left of those dreadful final years of her marriage. I had braced myself for the possibility of having been forgotten. But given the strength of our bond, I had not contemplated the possibility that my presence would make her recoil.

Over the next few days, I kept her company during meals. She was chipper and chatty some mornings, when she seemed curious about who I was and how I had wound up at her dining table. My answers were met with a blank stare. Meals were a sobering window into the process of memory loss. Coquis often recited poems out of the blue, their verses readily accessible. Virtually every day, she listed the names of her eight children in descending order of age, seeming eager to prove an ability to retain vital information. And she took pleasure in singing a vast repertoire of songs whose lyrics and melodies somehow escaped oblivion. I had all but given up on learning something new about her marriage. But one day, unexpectedly, she brought up Hernando in a string of sentences that was strikingly coherent, albeit untrue. "This house, with its thick walls, was built by Hernando before he died," she said. "Everything he built had a strong foundation."

Hernando passed away decades before my grandmother first laid eyes on Barichara, which has become a popular destination for retirees and tourists. I asked if she thought of Hernando often. "Of course!" she said. He'd built this home we were in, she repeated, noting the thickness of the white walls. Hernando had understood the value of a sturdy substructure, she said. I let the moment sink in, not even entertaining the possibility of setting the record straight. I was struck that as large chunks of her memory eroded, she had found a way to rewrite a dreadful chapter of the past. She told the same story, unprompted, the next day, marveling again at the girth of the walls, and this time adding that he had played a role in furnishing the living room with dark wooden rocking chairs. It struck me how differently we were going about making sense of the past. While I had seen value in uncovering difficult strands of my family history in order to make sense of my propensity for depression, Coquis's diminishing mind had seemingly taken a different approach common among people with dementia: constructing false memories that must have provided some solace.

During our final morning together, Coquis looked tired and didn't seem eager to chat, so we listened in silence to one of the playlists saved on her phone. She perked up at the first notes of a song that brought back memories of my father, who would belt out the lyrics annoyingly loudly during road trips: "Yo También Tuve 20 Años"—I too was 20 years old once—by Garzón y Collazos.

"I too was once 20, and a vagabond heart, I too had joys and profound disappointments," we sang in unison, and at last I felt a semblance of closeness to this vanishing ancestor sitting beside me, at once so familiar and impenetrable.

As I drove away, I mourned the fading bond with my sole living grandparent. As an immigrant, I have long felt a sense of rootlessness. Watching Coquis fade in slow motion amplified that. For so long, she had been the center of gravity of a clan of eight children and twenty-one grandchildren. Now, with much of the family scattered around the globe, there was no longer a place or matriarch to serve as home, to anchor the sprawling clan.

I felt inconsolably alone.

4 THE YAWANAWÁ

The Tribe That Sprang Back from the Brink of Extinction

SURELY A RESPONSIBLE ADULT WOULD intervene, I thought as I watched the scene unfold, itching to step in. Pekan Rasu, a jovial member of the Yawanawá tribe, was pouring ayahuasca into a bottle cap, standing before a gaggle of eager boys who looked to be between the ages of eight and ten.

"It's the first time they're drinking," he told me, flashing a mischievous grin. "They've been asking to try it."

Like altar boys waiting for Communion, the lanky kids approached Pekan Rasu solemnly and took turns gulping down a squirt of the bitter brew. Wincing from the taste, they walked away unsteadily and settled down near a roaring campfire.

The last glimmers of daylight were fading at Mushu Inu village, one of a constellation of riverside hamlets in a remote area of the Amazon rainforest, revealing a sky that would soon fill with stars. Someone nearby strummed a guitar as Pekan Rasu sat next to the children and began chanting in a low, raspy voice. The boys had been laughing and playing all afternoon, but now their eyes closed and they appeared to settle into a trance. One smiled broadly, seemingly lost in a state of rapture. Another jerked his chest back and forth restlessly. A third looked distressed until a couple of tears streamed down his cheek—then he seemed at peace. When I saw Mushu Inu, an elder the village is named after, walking toward us, I figured there would be a reckoning and a reprimand for Pekan Rasu. Surely these kids were too young to be drinking ayahuasca. But Pekan Rasu began chanting louder and proudly proclaimed to Mushu Inu: "*Entraram na força.*" They're in the zone. Mushu Inu took in the scene, nodded, smiled approvingly, and walked away. Evidently, there is no minimum drinking age for ayahuasca in this corner of the Amazon. That was the first of several jolting lessons I would learn during a ten-day stay with the Yawanawá.

∿∿ I had arrived the day before to Mushu Inu village, which lies on the banks of the Gregório River, primarily drawn by the prospect of drinking ayahuasca as close as possible to the birthplace of these rituals. But there was a second motivation. It had become clear that a core strand of my depression was a sense of dislocation from my family, a phenomenon I'd seen in the stories of countless people I had met on psychedelic retreats. Yet, in the Amazon basin, a cluster of communities have somehow managed to retain the type of tribal structures that were once the norm among humans and have now become something of a relic. I wanted to understand how they defied the forces that make so many contemporary families scattered and so many of us effectively tribeless.

In recent years, the Yawanawá has become an iconic tribe in the psychedelic renaissance, captivating outsiders with joyful music, exuberant nighttime ceremonies, and a remarkable comeback tale. They were on the brink of extinction by the end of the twentieth century, having been ravaged by disease, enslaved by rubber trappers, and co-opted by Christian missionaries who sought to ban their ritualistic use of mind-altering plants. In the early 1980s, when fewer than one hundred Yawanawá remained, tribal leaders led a rebellion against the missionaries, got out of the rubber business, and resurrected their traditional use of medicinal plants, chiefly ayahuasca. Around the turn of the century, the Yawanawá launched an annual festival at their oldest village, called New Hope, which attracts hundreds of people. This was the beginning of a spiritual revival that would become the tribe's main source of revenue and cultural relevance. Yawanawá delegations now travel across Brazil and to cities abroad to lead ayahuasca ceremonies. In recent years, village elders began hosting groups of visitors for *vivencias*, or immersions. The visits are promoted as a rare opportunity to partake in ancient spiritual traditions in one of the remotest and most pristine areas of the Amazon rainforest.

I signed up for one hoping it would help me piece together the complex history of the brew that had so radically altered my mood, outlook, and habits years before. I was enticed by the idea that I was stepping into a more sacred, authentic realm of the ayahuasca world, guided by the keepers of an ancient lineage. At a time when the Amazon was being destroyed at an astonishing rate, I hoped to find in the Yawanawá's story a glimmer of hope that had been distressingly absent in my coverage of Indigenous communities in Brazil. How did this tribe manage to evade ethnocide, win a seminal land rights battle, and draw devotees from around the world—all from tiny villages that lack electricity and plumbing?

〰〰 I'm a little embarrassed to admit that my Yawanawá immersion began with an Instagram ad. The algorithm gods had long since registered my interest in psychedelics, and one afternoon, I watched a video posted by Renata Caldas da Silva, a Brazilian woman who has been drinking ayahuasca for decades and who organizes trips to Indigenous villages. It featured a group of people in bathing suits, covered in a thin layer of greenish mud, dancing in front of a towering samaúma tree. A couple of clicks later, I was chatting with Renata on WhatsApp, where virtually all business is conducted in Brazil. She easily persuaded me to wire her $400 to secure my spot in the upcoming "Carnival retreat," billed as an ideal escape from the boozy, hedonistic hordes that overtake Brazilian cities in late February.

It took four flights to get to the nearest city with an airport, Cruzeiro do Sul, a dusty town that saw its heyday during the Amazon rubber boom at the end of the nineteenth century. During the final minutes of the flight, I looked out the window and saw what had become a grimly familiar scene after working in Brazil for more than four years: small gashes appear in a sea of emerald green, patches of barren land that eventually merge into an ever-expanding frontier wiping away teeming ecosystems in the world's largest rainforest to make room for raising cattle.

After landing, I met up with the other three passengers headed to Mushu Inu village for an anti-Carnival sojourn. Like me, they had embarked on this pilgrimage after clicking on an Instagram ad. Deise, an attorney from southern Brazil who teaches kundalini yoga on the side, was fulfilling a lifelong dream of traveling to the Amazon. The other two, Mariano and Karina, a couple from São Paulo, told us they had embarked on this adventure hoping to get guidance from a higher source on whether they should split up or find a way to mend their strained relationship.

In Cruzeiro do Sul, we boarded a van that zigzagged around potholes on a road bordered by cattle ranches. Two hours later, we reached the gateway to Yawanawá country: a muddy marina where small riverboats take turns picking up and dropping off passengers. After we got settled in ours, the skipper fired up the motor, which made an earsplitting whine, and propelled us away from the world of cars, cell phone service, and political banners and into the meandering muddy river.

The ride to the village took six hours as the overloaded boat fought against the current, maneuvering around shallow patches and protruding logs. Wading into a stretch of untainted rainforest in the Amazon evokes feelings of awe and helplessness. The cacophony of croaking frogs, buzzing insects, howling monkeys, and screeching birds is at once captivating and overwhelming.

Each Yawanawá village was built around an ancient samaúma tree.

They loom stoically over the unruly tangle of skinnier trees, vines, and shrubs. Among the oldest beings in the rainforest, samaúmas have borne quiet witness to cycles of life and death, abundance and privation, brutality and benevolence, some for more than a century.

We arrived at the village about an hour before sunset and were greeted by children and teenagers who swarmed the boat, eager to help carry our bags. We followed them past the houses nearest to the river and down a boardwalk to the open field where we would stay. Yawakashau, the cacique, or village chief, greeted us warmly alongside his wife, Maria Janete. They directed us to the center of the field, where a massive black pot was propped on two logs over a crackling campfire. Inside was a dark brown frothy brew with chunks of shredded ayahuasca vine, which had been boiling for more than twenty-four hours. Yawakashau said he had been cooking it personally to ensure we would have a sublime batch for the upcoming ceremonies. We were the inaugural guests in this section of the village, which consisted of a handful of wooden huts erected around a freshly cleared field that was roughly the size of a soccer stadium. Inspiration for the expansion of the village had come from a *miração*. It's a term longtime ayahuasca drinkers use to refer to something between a prophecy and a vision that happens during a particularly insightful trip. During a ceremony the year before, Yawakashau told us, the plants told him he would build this annex to host guests and to establish a cultural center that would help keep the tribe's culture and language—which Yawanawá children no longer speak fluently—alive for generations to come.

"When I closed my eyes I saw this terrain, in the shape of a circle, with houses all around," he said. Yawakashau pushed back on the prophetic voice, noting he didn't have much in the way of savings and how expensive it was to build anything in this remote stretch of the jungle. But the voice reassured him, saying: "This space is already yours." For good measure, it added a dazzling vision: one day, foreigners would be dancing under the stars during ayahuasca ceremonies Yawakashau would lead. Some would be enticed to stay to teach English to his children. For a split second, I tried on the vision, imagining what it would be like to go off the grid for a year or two to experience what life was like for our ancestors who lived in tribal communities. But that fantasy disintegrated as soon as we got a tour of the facilities. There was no running water in Mushu Inu. The lone shower facility in our area consisted of a large tub of water with a bucket, where I spotted a couple of tarantulas. Meals were cooked over a wood-fueled fire. Going to the bathroom meant walking down an unlit, narrow trail to a wooden cubicle that had a hole hovering over a barrel. This setup struck me as far from ideal for the explosive purging the body is prone to do under the influence of ayahuasca. But if I had come in search of ancient traditions, I would have to make do with ancient infrastructure.

〰 Just how long Indigenous people in the Amazon have been using mind-altering plants is a question that has puzzled and divided experts. Ayahuasca is prepared by boiling crushed chunks of an Amazonian vine called *Banisteriopsis caapi*—which wraps around trees in the rainforest in serpentlike formations—with the leaves of a shrubby plant called *Psychotria viridis*, or chacruna. The leaves contain the psychoactive compound, but when taken alone, an enzyme in the stomach neutralizes it. The vine, however, inhibits that metabolic process, inducing dramatic alterations in perception and sensations. Veteran ayahuasca makers often pray as they collect the vine and the leaves. And they cook it ritualistically over an open fire, inhaling the sweet vapor for hours and hours.

Jeremy Narby, a Canadian anthropologist who wrote a 1998 book about ayahuasca called *The Cosmic Serpent*, described Amazonian shamanism as an "academic discipline" that predates the most respected universities in the world by thousands of years. Shamans who trained with ayahuasca, he wrote, "hold the keys to a way of knowledge that they have practiced without interruption for at least five thousand years." Comparatively, he noted, "the universities of the Western world are less than nine hundred years old."

Esther Jean Langdon, a Tulane-trained anthropologist who has done extensive fieldwork with Amazonian tribes in Colombia, is convinced that ayahuasca has been used since prehistoric times. "We're talking about ten thousand years, at least," she told me during an interview at her home in southern Brazil. But other academics who have studied Amazonian societies and customs have pushed back on those assertions in recent years. They argue that ayahuasca rituals have likely been around for no more than five hundred years.

Steve Beyer, a religious studies scholar from the United States who spent years studying shamanism in Peru and wrote a book called *Singing to the Plants*, has criticized the romanticization of ayahuasca as a medicine that has been around for thousands of years. "In an attempt to legitimize ayahuasca use, its proponents invoke the culturally resonant trope of millennia-old Indigenous wisdom," Beyer wrote in a 2012 essay titled "On the Origins of Ayahuasca." He added that it supports "the odd affectation of European colonialism that Indigenous people are *without history*—that unlike Europeans, they are unchanging in their isolation and innocence." Beyer argues that ayahuasca's origin story is likely to be no more than a few centuries old and likely has a surprisingly mundane explanation: to treat children with parasitic illnesses, Indigenous people in the Amazon turned to plant remedies that induced purging. Another prominent challenger of the millennial theory is Bernd Brabec de Mori, a cultural anthropologist and musicologist at the University of Innsbruck in Austria, who lived in a Peruvian Indigenous community for several years. De Mori says that ayahuasca appears to have become widespread along the Amazon basin only after colonization, as Jesuit missions and rubber camps created more links and exchanges among tribes. Evgenia Fotiou, a cultural anthropologist in the United States who studies shamanism and ayahuasca tourism, says she would be surprised if ayahuasca was being brewed more than four hundred years ago. But regardless of its antiquity, she said, modern traditions are unlikely to bear much resemblance to the earliest ones. "Even if they did use these plants thousands of years ago, most likely they did not use them the same way they use them today."

∿∿∿ The oldest written accounts of ayahuasca ceremonies were recorded by Jesuit priests in the eighteenth century. They describe the rituals in foreboding terms, perhaps unsurprisingly given that the Catholic Church was on a mission to expand its influence in the New World. In 1737, Pablo Maroni, a Jesuit priest who watched an ayahuasca ritual near the Napo River, a tributary to the Amazon, penned a dispatch calling the brew "an intoxicating potion ingested for divination and other purposes . . . which deprives one of his senses and, at times, of his life."

I was eager to see where Yawanawá elders would land on the question of antiquity and whether they had their own theory of when exactly these rituals began. Several suggested I speak to Kateyuve Yawanawá, a Pagé, or trained medicine man, who was described to me as something of the tribe's unofficial historian. He lived in a village called Yawaraní, about an hour down the river, and was known by his nickname, Pai Nani. I imagined Pai Nani would be imposing and regal. But when we were introduced, I was struck by his slumped shoulders, aloof manner, and easygoing nature. When I tried to pin him down on a time for an interview, he demurred, seeming uninterested in making a concrete commitment. But when we finally sat down one afternoon, he talked for hours, never once bothering to check the time or signal impatience. Pai Nani patiently answered my questions as I sought to nail down a clear time line of the tribe's recent history. But it soon became evident that he deemed it an unimportant question and that he didn't share my preoccupation with dates and other means of tracking time imposed on Indigenous communities by white people.

Pai Nani's eyes widened with enthusiasm, though, when I asked about the origin of ayahuasca. He told me it dated to "time immemorial," a period when a benevolent king ruled the world. There was no death then, so people had little to fear and much time to learn from their mistakes. But everything changed one day when the king died suddenly. Having never had to deal with a lifeless body, the community was terrified—and stumped. There was a vigorous debate about what to do with it.

"Should we bury him?" one relative asked, according to Pai Nani.

Lacking a better idea, that's what they did. A few days after the death, a cousin who was close to the king, and who missed him dearly, visited the burial site. He was surprised to find a tangle of vines and plants that had sprouted from the plot. The cousin went home and, giving in to a sudden bout of sleepiness, collapsed into his hammock.

"His cousin came to him in his dreams and told him that all those plants were medicinal," Pai Nani said, telling the story more like a history lesson than a legend. The king then delivered sobering news: "From here on out, every human being who will live will also die, like me," Pai Nani said. "During life, there will be lots of illnesses, and these medicines will cure them."

In subsequent dreams, the king's cousin began getting detailed guidance on how to use plants medicinally, becoming the first Pagé in the Amazon, Pai Nani said. But it became apparent to him that penetrating the world of sacred plants, where spirits can be called upon to perform cures and curses, was no easy task. It required putting oneself through long periods of privation and sacrifice. That was the beginning of the tradition of dieting with plants, a custom that many tribes in the Amazon follow to this day to train plant medicine practitioners. The process entails spending months, sometimes even years, in social isolation, abstaining from sex and alcohol and surviving on very little food. Dieting tests the mettle and discipline of aspiring shamans, weeding out the curious from the resolute. Over time, plant spirits begin revealing their knowledge and bestowing their power to the latter, who become something of a conduit between the realm of mortals and that of spirits.

"You can speak to them just like I'm speaking to you," Pai Nani told me. "They have things to tell you."

〰〰 Pai Nani and other Yawanawá Pagés trace their lineage to Antô-nio Luiz Pekuti, who was among the Yawanawá elders who brokered contact with non-Indigenous people early in the 1900s. It was a pe-riod of upheaval and bloodshed remembered as the era of *correrias*, or being constantly on the run. The Yawanawá were under siege from Peruvian rubber tappers and at war with neighboring tribes. Families were constantly in mourning as smallpox and the flu ripped through the community. The deluge of existential threats made families put childbearing on hold.

"When girls had their first menstruation, they gave them medicine to make them infertile," Pai Nani told me. "They wanted to be able to pick up and run without much worry."

I imagined that Pagés would have been performing healing rituals nonstop in those days. But Pai Nani said that back then, spiritual leaders like Antônio Luiz, who was his uncle, were more like warriors and sorcerers than healers. The mysterious powers of the plant spir-its were used to put curses on rivals, to seduce desirable women, and to gain the upper hand in territorial conflicts.

"He took the lives of many people," Pai Nani told me nonchalantly. "It's easier to do evil. It's like hitting someone. It's easy to injure a person, but it's hard to cure them."

I was stunned. Ayahuasca is marketed today as a shortcut to happi-ness, a means to get ten years' worth of therapy in a couple of nights. It's described as a benevolent feminine energy that heals and soothes and comforts. But as I dug a bit deeper into how Indigenous people used and viewed its powers, I soon realized that Pai Nani's account was not an aberration. Langdon, the anthropologist who studied tribes in Colombia, including the Cofán and the Siona, said the sha-mans she observed for years described gaining access to a shadowy realm she called "the other side." It's a dimension inhabited by evil and benign spirits who can be called upon to wreak havoc or heal. "The other side is an animated universe that actually impacts our daily life," she explained. Earthly shamans who negotiate access to the other side can deliver curses and miracles—and often they end up trading in both. Fotiou, the cultural anthropologist who conducted extensive fieldwork in the Iquitos region of Peru between 2003 and 2007, said she was struck by how differently tourists and shamans understood ayahuasca. The former spoke about sublime healing journeys. The latter were in a never-ending battle against sorcery that has only escalated with the growing financial incentive to serve ayahuasca to foreigners. "They all talk about how there are these wars going on in the spiritual realm with other shamans, and they're all trying to get power," Fotiou told me. Among local people, she said, ayahuasca is still regarded as a healing tool, "but usually to heal sorcery."

〜〜 The rubber industry in the Amazon, which went into overdrive during World War II, strained the Yawanawá's culture by introducing capitalism, booze, and coercive labor. A new threat emerged in the 1970s when missionaries from the New Tribes Mission—an American Christian evangelical group bent on converting Indigenous people—moved in with the Yawanawá. The first wave of missionaries, who were Brazilian, had been welcomed. But when young American missionary couples joined them, things grew tense. The Americans were horrified by the rituals with ayahuasca, which they deemed demonic, and sought to impose a rigid schedule of study and playtime on a community that had long had an elastic sense of time. "You know Americans," Pai Nani told me. "If you don't play by their rules, you're in the wrong."

Things came to a head one day in the early 1980s when one of the Americans, a young man named Miguel, told young Yawanawá children playing soccer that they had to stop because the schedule indicated they ought to be doing something else. When the children resisted, Miguel brandished a gun. That incensed Yawanawá leaders, who decided that the missionaries had overstayed their welcome.

"The next day, we told them they had to leave," Pai Nani said. "We threw their things in a boat, and they left."

The departure of the missionaries in the early 1980s coincided with a period of political transformation in Brazil that would have profound consequences for Indigenous rights. The era of military rule, during which Brazil's leaders sought to industrialize the Amazon and push tribal communities into urban areas, was coming to an ignominious end. The 1988 constitution, which cemented the return to democracy after twenty-one years of despotic rule, recognized the rights of Indigenous people to their cultural heritage and over their ancestral lands. The Yawanawá became among the first tribes to get official recognition of their claim to almost five hundred thousand acres of the rainforest—part of a patchwork of Indigenous territories that makes up nearly 13 percent of Brazil's landmass.

With this victory came a sobering realization of what the Yawanawá had lost during the past tumultuous decades. Only the elderly spoke their native language fluently. Playful rituals known as *brincadeiras*, which had been handed down from generation to generation, had become a faint memory for just a few. And crucially, the devotion to the plant world as a catalyst for spiritual enlightenment and healing had been all but lost. Only two elders, known as Yawá and Tatá, had continued to brew ayahuasca, and their rites had become infrequent and clandestine, especially when missionaries lived in their village.

"We were left practically without culture," Mushu Inu told me one morning as we walked along a trail flanked by towering açaí trees. "We had it, but it hadn't been practiced in so long."

In an effort to resurrect old customs, young Yawanawá leaders asked Tatá and Yawá to bring back the grueling plant diets that turn ordinary people into plant whisperers and miracle makers. Pai Nani was among the handful of early disciples, along with his childhood friend Bira Brasil Yawanawá. When their training was complete, Bira, who became one of the tribe's leaders, made a couple of radical decisions. Henceforth, he decreed, ayahuasca rituals would be used only to heal, never to harm. And drinking ayahuasca would no longer be restricted to medicine men. Ceremonies would be led by men who had undergone extensive training through dieting, forging a deep connection to the plants. But anyone could drink. While the ceremonies of yore had featured only chanting, the new ones included drums and guitars, which gave a modern flair to traditional songs. And ecstatic dancing became a fixture of these rituals, making them feel more like parties than spiritual rites.

I felt a pang of disappointment upon learning just how modern these contemporary rituals were. It meant that I had been alive longer than Yawanawá ayahuasca ceremonies have existed in their current form. So much for partaking in ancient, authentic rites.

The following night, during our first ayahuasca ceremony, I drank a small serving and decided I would be more of an observer than a participant. After everyone was served, most participants joined hands in a circle and began walking clockwise, chanting a series of prayers intended to deter evil spirits and raise the group's collective energy. About an hour later, Pekan Rasu, wearing a massive feather headdress, chanted a wistful song. When he was done, instruments came out and fueled sets of long, frenetic melodies bracketed by chants of "*Pura alegria!*" Just joy. Feeling more sleepy than joyful, I slipped into my tent after 3:00 a.m., but struggled to get proper rest because the music and hollering carried on uninterrupted until dawn.

Late the next morning, I sought out Pekan Rasu. I was curious to learn more about the pageantry of the night before. And I wanted to delicately broach the subject of the drinking age. Despite having stayed up all night singing and dancing, Pekan Rasu was brimming with energy. He told me he learned how to run ceremonies from his father, Yawá, one of the two Pagés in the tribe who kept spiritual rituals alive during the era of the rubber tappers and the missionaries. Yawá, he told me, had died in 2018 at the age of 106 and had remained remarkably sharp and healthy until the end, partaking in ceremonies as they morphed into increasingly elaborate, gleeful, and communal affairs. He explained that the chanting circle at the beginning of the ceremony re-creates a myth about how human beings

made an evolutionary leap that distinguished them from other animals, a turning point reenacted with guttural grunts. Songs then
get more melodic and playful. Some make sense of the mystery of
romantic attraction, exploring how people flirt and ultimately form
long-term pairings. Others address the visceral bonds between parents and their children. The halfway point of the ceremony, when
the Pagé sings alone, is a crucial moment, Pekan Rasu said. "I ask
the ancestral keepers of the medicine, the spirits, to be among us, to
guide us, to take care of us."

When I asked about children drinking ayahuasca, I expected
Pekan Rasu would be defensive or perhaps a bit embarrassed. He was
neither. He said it's wrong to think about ayahuasca as an intoxicant.
Rather, he said, it's a "medicine that teaches." His sister-in-law Maria Janete, who had been listening to us, weighed in to say she had
initially been apprehensive when her daughter Amanda asked to try
her first sips when she was about eight. But she soon discovered that
children who drank from an early age become more self-aware and
loving. "It transforms how they act," she said. "They apologize more
often" when they have upset someone. "They hug more. They express
gratitude more." After hearing this, I observed the behavior of the
children and teenagers at the village. A few things stood out. They
always seemed to be on the lookout for opportunities to help adults
with tasks big and small. There was a reverence especially for the elderly that seemed to undergird every interaction. While I snuck away
alone to eat snacks I had brought, I noticed the kids were predisposed
to sharing. And I came to see their devotion to playing music together
throughout the day as a glue that kept people in the village connected.

During the third and final ceremony at Mushu Inu, I helped myself
to a bigger dose and committed to being more of a participant than
a detached observer. Soon after the chanting circle began churning,
I slipped in and locked arms with two men. I added my voice to the
incantation, initially softly and hesitantly, then gaining confidence and
volume with each step. A few minutes in, I gave in to the electrifying
feeling of being in lockstep with other people. There was magic and

depth in this ritual that had looked so befuddling and basic a few nights before.

When the chanting phase ended and Pekan Resu sang to invoke the spirits, I sat by the fire and felt tears pooling in my closed eyes. Suddenly, a string of words pierced my thoughts: *You strayed from your tribe.* I sat with these words for a few minutes, allowing them to play over and over in my head. What began as a mantra turned into a taunt that gave way to memory. I took stock of how loosely I had stayed in touch with my parents and my sisters after leaving home for college at eighteen. I reflected on how often I had moved since then, always in the pursuit of new job titles and adventures. I considered with deep curiosity my persistent urge to lurch forward, farther away from the point of origin, realizing I had never reflected on the trade-offs of a series of decisions that had added up to a profoundly lonely existence. I made a note of how geographically splintered my core and extended family had become as cousins, aunts, and uncles, for various reasons, opted to build lives far from Colombia. A majority of us, it seemed, had given up on our homeland and let the bonds of blood fray. I allowed the sadness of that thought to sink in, avoiding the temptation to shift gears to a different idea. Then a new set of words crystallized: *You can rebuild your tribe.* I sat with them, wondering what that could look like. Would the idea seem ludicrous when daylight came? Or was this an invitation I could accept?

Lacking a clear answer, I found myself springing up from the floor and joining a group of people facing the musicians. The pounding of the drums gave me a reprieve from melancholic thoughts as I slipped into the choreography, taking two steps forward and two steps back. I stared up at the sky, again brimming with stars, and spotted a constellation of fireflies that seemed to be twinkling on and off in sync with the music. I marveled at how light and unburdened I suddenly felt, at how dramatically getting up to dance had lifted my mood. This was not my tribe, I understood. But for one night, for a magical few hours, I gave myself permission to feel the power and strength of being in a community of lives and fates that are tightly bound, securely interwoven.

5   HOLY AYAHUASCA

THE PULL TOWARD A SPIRITUAL path first came to Alex Polari in a prison cell, after years of isolation and brutal torture.

He was among the militant leftists of his generation in Brazil who joined guerrilla groups and took up arms to topple the despotic military leaders who ruled the country for twenty-one years, starting in 1964. Their cause had been a righteous one, Alex told me, but the crucible of incarceration changed the nature of his revolutionary zeal and brought a realization that would alter the trajectory of his life.

"I don't disown everything we did, the radicalism, the armed fight, but the time had come to launch a revolution within," he said. "Without that, it's hard for you to change the broader world."

When he left prison in 1979, in the waning years of the dictatorship, Alex considered embarking on a pilgrimage to India. He yearned to find a contemplative practice, perhaps a guru, ideally thousands of miles from his homeland, to make peace with the sacrifice and trauma of the past decade. Before he could pack his bags, a friend and fellow revolutionary who had moved to the Amazon after being released from prison told Alex about a mysterious spiritual tradition called Santo Daime that was gaining followers and raising eyebrows in Rio Branco, a small city in the state of Acre, in the northwest corner of the Amazon. Alex had recently purchased video equipment, intending to break into documentary making. But on hearing about the nascent religion taking root on the outskirts of the Amazon, he decided to explore it. India would have to wait.

What he found in Acre would forever change his life and his outlook and turned him into a leading figure in the quest to legalize the use of ayahuasca in Brazil and expand its appeal well beyond South America.

Alex learned that Santo Daime had been founded by a Black illiterate rubber tapper called Raimundo Irineu Serra, who began participating in Indigenous ayahuasca rituals starting around 1914. During one of his early ceremonies, Raimundo, who became known as Mestre Irineu, had a powerful *miração*, or vision. He reported having seen a full moon drifting toward him, transporting a celestial being. He came to recognize the being as the Queen of the Forest, an embodiment of the Virgin Mary. The Queen, Mestre Irineu would later tell friends and followers, commanded him to establish a new religious movement that would blend Indigenous rituals, Christian liturgy, and African spiritual traditions.

It was an outlandish claim that could have easily subjected Mestre Irineu to ridicule. Here was a man of humble origins, the grandson of slaves—Brazil only outlawed slavery in 1888—proclaiming to have found a direct line to Jesus and the Virgin Mary by imbibing a psychoactive Indigenous brew that had long been vilified by Christian leaders. If this vision were to take hold, Brazil was the ideal place to propagate it; the country has for centuries been an incubator for several syncretic religious practices that draw from the traditions of its vastly diverse population.

In the years following the supposed prophecy, Mestre Irineu led an ordinary life, making a living as a military police officer in the Amazon. By the 1930s, he began leading small services with ayahuasca out of his simple home, and a congregation that began with a handful of people started to multiply.

Mestre Irineu told disciples that celestial beings had chosen him to impart profound truths and pragmatic life advice to human beings at a tipping point for humanity. Their guidance, he explained, was transmitted through hymns that were channeled from the astral plane. The first song that came to him was titled *"Lua Branca,"* White Moon. It is a devotional ode to the moon, which becomes a symbol of the grace and radiance of the Virgin Mary. A recurring line in the song is *"Daime o perdão."* In Portuguese, *daime* means "give me," and *perdão* means "forgiveness." As more hymns came to him, and later to some of his disciples, *"Daime"* became a recurring plea. Give me faith, give me strength, give me love—so the religion came to be called Santo Daime. The ayahuasca brewed for their services, called *trabalhos*, or works, became known simply as Daime.

What began as a tiny congregation in Rio Branco grew slowly over the years and eventually splintered into a handful of sects amid personal and liturgical rifts. Santo Daime elders became known as *padrinhos* and *madrinhas*, godfathers and godmothers, which spoke to the familial and tight-knit nature of Daime clans. Leading figures within the tradition began recording their own hymn collections, which became an ever-growing and evolving body of liturgy.

Some popular hymns are stern, warning about sin and the emptiness of a life devoid of faith. Many are playful, often packing multiple strands of meaning in verses that appear simple at first glance. A prominent theme is the importance of learning to cultivate love and devotion: to God, to kin, to neighbors and strangers. Several Daime songs read like poems that pay tribute to the beauty and wonder of the natural world. One of Mestre Irineu's hymns urges his followers to refrain from gossip, a tall order in Brazil.

Another feature that makes Santo Daime incongruous with the culture in which it emerged is the rigidity of its rituals. Brazilians are notoriously unpunctual, noncommittal, and improvisational. Yet Santo Daime demands meticulous adherence to the rules and traditions of

works. Santo Daime initiates wear formal white uniforms to ceremonies. Men don blue ties, and women wear black bow ties. Men
and women sit in opposing sides of Santo Daime churches, some of
which are shaped like stars.

Twice a month, Daimistas gather for meditative rituals known as
works of concentration. After drinking Daime and reciting a few prayers,
congregants sit in silence and are instructed to empty the mind of
day-to-day thoughts and tap into a higher state of consciousness.

Holy Mass works, held on the first Monday of every month, are
intended to assist the souls of people who have died to transcend.

Then there are the Bailados, or dancing works, which are performed
on special occasions. The ritual is an overnight marathon of endur-
ance during which Daimistas sing and dance for as long as ten hours
while drinking Daime. They follow a simple choreography, taking two
steps to the right, then two steps to the left, in perfect synchrony.
Daime leaders say the choreography creates a unified frequency that
enables individuals to grow and transcend as a collective.

It goes without saying that to outsiders—even enthusiasts of entheogenic plants—Santo Daime rituals can seem bizarre—cultish,
even. Mindful of that, Daimistas, as a foundational rule, have long
refrained from proselytizing. Newcomers who want to attend a ceremony are typically screened carefully to assess their state of mind
and motivations. Many people who participate in Daime rituals for
the first time never come back. Others warm up to its teachings and
stoic traditions slowly. Then there are the instant converts, people
like Alex Polari.

〰〰 Mestre Irineu had been dead for a little over a decade when
Alex first traveled to the Amazon to visit a Santo Daime congregation run by one of the founder's leading disciples, Padrinho Sebastião
Mota de Melo. While he gathered footage for a documentary, Alex
was invited to participate in a ceremony. Soon after gulping down the
bitter, sludgy brew, Alex had a powerful *miração*.

"Everything made sense, and it left me without any doubts about the nature of reality," Alex said. "This was what I had been looking for."

The experience radically expanded the bounds of his perception, Alex told me. It became evident to him that all humans are endowed with God's divine essence. The Daime offered a shortcut to tap into that ethereal nature and harness its power for individual and collective transformation, Alex said. But getting there demanded a grueling amount of introspection. In *The Religion of Ayahuasca*, a book Alex published in 2010, he compared that process to the work of a gardener who must intentionally water and tend to the seeds he wants to sprout. That required a lot of weeding. "My consciousness was a real junkyard," Alex wrote. "A junkyard with aspirations of becoming a sanctuary."

Soon after Alex became a Santo Daime initiate, elders in the movement asked him to help them navigate an existential challenge. Word about Santo Daime had begun spreading beyond the jungle, attracting spiritual seekers from large Brazilian cities and from neighboring countries. And government officials had grown concerned. The mass murder–suicide involving more than nine hundred members of the cult led by Jim Jones in Guyana was fresh in people's minds. So in 1982, a delegation from the Brazilian government led by an army colonel was dispatched to a new Santo Daime community that had been established deep in the rainforest.

"Everyone thought they were going to stumble into a cult of fanatics," said Alex, who served as a member of the commission. "We endured a lot of stigma and persecution."

The members of the commission were welcomed with open arms, Alex said, and appeared to leave persuaded that Daimistas were healthy, serious about their spiritual practice, and harmless. But just a few years later, in 1985, as Brazil's dictatorship came to a sputtering halt, the federal health regulatory agency issued a decree banning the use of ayahuasca. By then, Daimistas had formed a handful of residential communes in the country, including one Alex established near Visconde de Mauá, a bucolic village in the mountains near Rio de Janeiro. Daimistas and allies from other religious groups that had adopted ayahuasca as a sacrament put up a fight. They persuaded the government to establish an interdisciplinary commission to study the religious use of ayahuasca. The group, which included government officials, anthropologists, and psychiatrists, issued a detailed report in 1987 recognizing the use of ayahuasca as an ancient spiritual tradition and recommended that religious groups be allowed to make and consume the brew. The report led the health agency to lift its ban.

But the legality of ayahuasca was far from a settled matter. In the early 1990s, a series of scandals involving Santo Daime made headlines, sparking a national debate about the safety of the rituals and the integrity of its leaders. Much of the outcry was driven by allegations by a church member, Alicia Castilla. She accused Alex and other leaders of his community of brainwashing her teenage daughter, who wound up living in the commune Alex established when she was fourteen. In a book titled *Santo Daime: Fanaticism and Brainwashing*, Alicia claimed that Santo Daime leaders had lured severely sick people, including AIDS patients, with false hopes that they could be cured by drinking Daime. Some Daimistas, she asserted, charged thousands of dollars to foreign patients desperate for a Hail Mary. Alicia recounted the story of a young man who had joined the church, became psychologically unstable, and died by suicide by jumping into an open fire. She noted that a Frenchwoman who had spent time in a Santo Daime community had returned home severely depressed and killed herself.

In a lengthy written rebuttal at the time, Alex defended the church and asserted that Santo Daime was not in the business of curing illness. Desperate, despondent people often turn to spiritual communities, he noted, and Daimistas felt a responsibility to do right by those who turned to their churches. "Without a doubt, in these current times, practicing charity has become a high-risk endeavor," he wrote. "We have a spiritual obligation to care for all the people who come to us."

In the years that followed, government officials and members of ayahuasca churches felt it was necessary to set clearer rules for the religious use of the brew and to clarify the extent to which it could be used as a therapeutic tool. In 2004, the National Council on Drug Policy, a federal agency, established yet another multidisciplinary group tasked with drafting a set of principles. In a report issued two years later, the government committee recognized the religious use of ayahuasca as an ancestral practice worthy of legal protection. But it laid out strict parameters informed by an emerging consensus that robust safeguards were needed to prevent abuses and malpractice given how powerfully and suddenly ayahuasca could induce profound changes in behavior.

For starters, the commission decreed that ayahuasca should not be commercialized and took a dim view of its use as a tourism draw. Ayahuasca churches, it opined, should be measured in the content they post online, abstaining from promising "miraculous cures" or "dramatic personal transformations." Committee members acknowledged that people who are ill and suffering often find solace in faith, which made it hard to outright ban healing rituals using ayahuasca. But it noted that *curanderismo*—traditional healing rituals led by people without traditional medical credentials—is illegal in Brazil. Any therapeutic use outside religious settings should be limited to authorized scientific studies, the committee said. Finally, it called on groups to carefully screen first-time participants and subject them to an interview to prevent its use among "people with a history of mental illness."

~~~ I arrived for my screening interview at Alex Polari's commune in the mountains around dusk on a Wednesday in early December, about half an hour before a major dancing work honoring the Virgin Mary was set to begin. The ground was soggy from torrential rain earlier in the day, so I hopped over muddy patches as Marcelo, a tall, burly member of the community, guided me to the wooden, star-shaped church. The centerpiece of an idyllic residential com-

munity home to some forty individuals, the church has a star-shaped wooden altar in the center. Hanging from the cone-shaped ceiling are strings of white, frilly decorations and golden cutouts of moons, suns, and stars.

Marcelo led me to a small, cluttered room in the back, pulled out a clipboard, and began asking questions. After recording basic biographical details, he asked whether I was "stable and satisfied" in my profession. "It depends on the day," I told him with a smile. He asked if I had been hospitalized for psychiatric problems. I told him I had not. He asked whether I belonged to a religion. Nope. He wanted to know if I had experienced mystical phenomena. I offered a muddled response. Satisfied, Marcelo gave me the green light to participate in the ritual.

As the last glimmer of daylight receded, I spotted Alex and his wife, Sonia, as they arrived in the church, and introduced myself. I had been in touch with Alex for nearly a year about a possible visit. He had been cordial, but noncommittal. Before extending a formal invitation, he set one condition: I could visit as part of research for a book, but not for an article in the newspaper. Santo Daime, he made clear, prefers to stay out of the headlines. Alex is a towering figure in the ayahuasca world, having played a key role in fighting for its legalization in Brazil and abroad. But he deliberately keeps a low profile, abstaining from social media and the psychedelics conference circuit. He greeted me warmly, speaking in a low, gentle voice. As I took stock of this mild-mannered elderly man who keeps a long white beard, it was hard to imagine he had once been an armed rebel.

As congregants trickled in for the work, I noted that women wore glittering tiaras and colorful ribbons that swayed from their shoulders. On the men's side, I spotted a handful of foreigners, including a gray-haired man from Switzerland, an Italian who was becoming a Santo Daime initiate that night, and a young man from Oregon. When the ceremony was about to begin, a stern-looking man approached to guide me to my assigned spot for the evening: a rectangle demarcated on the floor that was about three feet by one foot, where

I would be confined to dance for the next eight hours or so. I later learned this man was the *fiscal*, or enforcer of the rules of the ritual. After about thirty minutes of reciting Our Fathers and Hail Marys, Alex walked to the area where the Daime is served and began filling shot glasses as men and women lined up separately to receive the sacrament. After the first of several servings, the singing began with the first song in Mestre Irineu's 130-hymn collection, which is called *The Cross*. Slightly nauseated by the drink, I struggled to keep pace despite the simplicity of the dance, two small steps to the left, two small steps to the right. Veteran Daimistas kept the beat, shaking small maracas with admirable precision. I was awed by the vigor of their singing and dancing, which seemed to strengthen with each song. Worshippers in their sixties and seventies displayed extraordinary stamina as I began feeling light-headed with fatigue and a slight discomfort in my feet began morphing into outright pain. As my unease grew, my mind was flooded with judgmental thoughts. *Cult! This clearly is a cult! Hours of rigid dancing while drinking ayahuasca can't be healthy! Children! They have children around who should be asleep in quiet rooms! Blatant cultural appropriation!* One hymn in particular, about the death of Jesus, made me balk for its flagrant anti-Semitism. "He suffered on the cross / He was imprisoned and tied up / It was the Jews that killed him / There in Judea everyone was pardoned." *Jesus Fucking Christ!*

Sometime past midnight, three cups of Daime in, somehow, inexplicably, the crescendo of discomfort came to an end, like a wave that reached its peak and crashed. I hadn't fundamentally changed my mind about the ideas that had surfaced with such acidity just hours before. But I had somehow managed to quiet a turbulent thought stream and enter a state of surrender. As I swayed right and left, I gazed at the decorative moons, stars, and suns dangling from the ceiling. They seemed full of life. I gave up on following the lyrics in my hymnbook and simply took in the beat, one cog in a swaying circle of souls. As dawn neared and only a handful of songs in the hymnbook remained unsung, I took a seat on a bench in the back of the room to rest my legs. The *fiscal* approached and urged me to get back on my feet. The last hymns were important, he stressed, friendly but stern. A few hours earlier, I would have put up a fight. But I acquiesced, returned to my small dancing rectangle, and found unexpected reserves of energy that overrode my exhaustion. When it was finally over, Alex approached and asked whether I had "entered into the force."

I understood that to mean having crossed into another dimension, having made the leap into a new level of understanding and cognition that had the potential to radically upend worldviews and mindsets. I had not, not even close, and I couldn't decide whether that left me feeling relieved or disappointed.

Before traveling to Visconde de Mauá, I had read everything I could get my hands on about the history of the Daime and found myself feeling fascinated and wary in equal measure. I had heard several Daime initiates describe having stumbled into the spiritual community as though they were being drawn by an invisible, unyielding force. Converts report feeling that they've been recruited by a higher power, a force they come to respect and revere, that is amassing an army of humans to shift the course of humanity. Once enlisted, they say they undergo an arduous process of introspection and transformation that then creates ripples, changing relationships and ultimately communities.

One striking initiation story came from William Barnard, a professor of religious studies at Southern Methodist University in Dallas, who wrote a book about his journey as a Santo Daime initiate. William had been a devoted follower of Swami Muktananda, the Indian yoga guru, and had a long-standing meditation practice when he first heard about Santo Daime in 2004. After a few years of attending Daime works, William said he felt a calling, clear as a lightning bolt, to become a *fardado*, or initiate. "It wasn't a rational thing," William told me. "I got this really strong inner message, like someone had grabbed me by the scruff of the neck and it was really clear: I'm doing it."

In his book *Liquid Light*, William describes Daime rituals as exhausting, often pushing people to the limits of what seems possible to endure physically. The reward, he writes, is having *mirações,* moments of incandescent clarity and joy that he says are experienced by accessing spiritual realms. "We can merge with Beings of Light and be granted a glimpse of the purity and profundity of their diamond-like, love-suffused vision of the cosmos," William wrote in his book. "Our physical / emotional ailments can be healed via the shimmering and exceedingly potent crystalline presence of compassionate spiritual 'doctors.'"

I have long struggled to make sense of such exuberant accounts, which are common among people who have been drinking ayahuasca for years. Sometimes I'm inclined to think they're merely hallucinations. Yet it's enticing to be open to the possibility that such realms not only exist but are accessible to mere mortals. What is evident is that people who report having these experiences regularly find them life-altering. When I asked William how drinking Daime for years had changed him, he didn't have to think hard. It had sharpened his mind, he told me, and made him more resilient. But the change that mattered most, he added, was one his late wife saw. "My wife said Santo Daime was what made me open my heart," he said. "It increased my capacity to love."

〜〜 A couple of days after the work, I returned to the community, called Céu da Montanha, to interview Alex. It was the end of a *feitio,* a weeklong festivity during which the community comes together to brew copious amounts of Daime. Alex told me that the growing global appeal of ayahuasca happened organically starting in the 1980s. "It was very spontaneous," he said, describing how a trickle of foreigners who found their way to sleepy Santo Daime communities grew into dozens of congregations abroad. "They would take Daime home, share it with people, and it started taking off," he said. "Suddenly, you had all these blond, blue-eyed Europeans singing in perfect Portuguese."

I asked him how he saw the boom of ayahuasca beyond the confines of Santo Daime and other similarly rigorous groups that strive to be largely inconspicuous. Did the increasingly flashy and high-priced retreat industry give him pause? Alex smiled and took a while before answering. He told me he had come to believe that sacred plants with the power to change minds and soften hearts are imbued with agency and intelligence. By spreading well beyond the Amazon, picking up converts from a broad cross section of humanity, the plants may be signaling a sense of urgency and distress about the state of the earth and its most destructive inhabitants, Alex said.

"They show us that there are things that are deeply wrong in our planet: everything from the climate crisis, social problems, environmental degradation, runaway capitalism," he said. "We're in a crisis of civilization."

Alex, who speaks in careful and deliberate language, told me he feels "a certain terror" when he contemplates the world humans are creating. If there's an off-ramp, he said, it will require changing human behavior quickly and on a massive scale. "We're in a race against time," he said. "The way I see it, plants, especially ayahuasca, might be the only shortcut to reach an expansion of consciousness that will be required to change."

The dilemma, Alex said, is that movements like Santo Daime have always expanded slowly and deliberately. There's no plan to change that. So the plants may be looking for bolder actors. That possibility gives him both hope and pause.

"I'm in favor of this movement expanding more and more each day, and of more people having insights, whether in religious or non-religious settings," he said. "But the way it's unfolding is very chaotic, very bewildering."

2

~~~~~~~~~~

THE WILD WEST OF PSYCHEDELIC RETREATS IN LATIN AMERICA

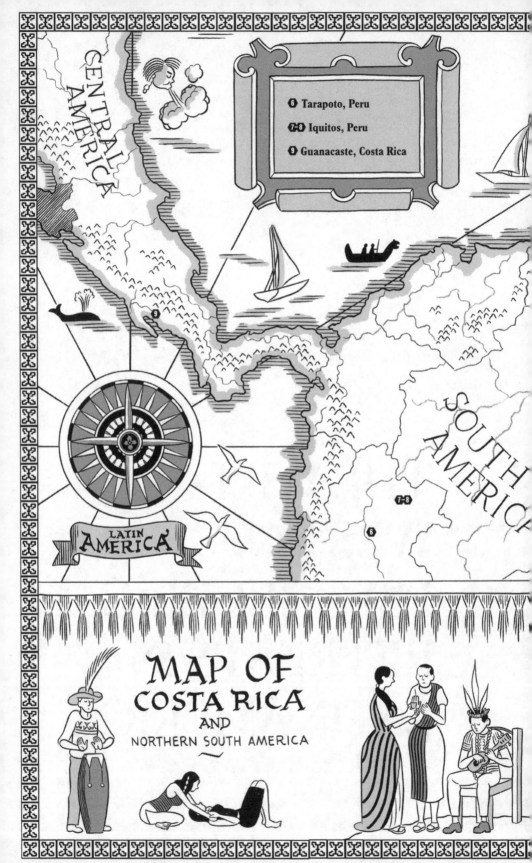

6 Tarapoto, Peru

7-8 Iquitos, Peru

9 Guanacaste, Costa Rica

CENTRAL AMERICA

SOUTH AMERICA

LATIN AMERICA

MAP OF COSTA RICA
AND
NORTHERN SOUTH AMERICA

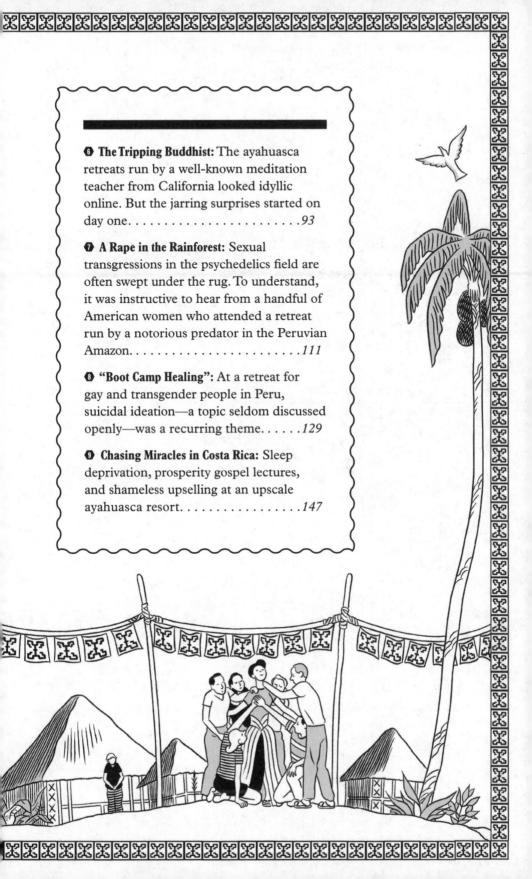

6   THE TRIPPING BUDDHIST

THE RED FLAGS WERE THERE from the start, in the hold-harmless agreement participants were required to sign on the first day of our Lotus Vine Journeys retreat. Several of us exchanged nervous chuckles and discreetly raised eyebrows as we scanned the document at the outdoor dining area of the Pumarinri Amazon Lodge, an upscale eco resort on the edge of the Amazon rainforest in Peru.

"During the course of a 14 day retreat, if a participant's behavior presents a threat to the safety of themselves or others, we reserve the right to physically restrain the guest and/or expel them from the retreat," the form advised. "Guest restraint will be conducted as gently as possible and with respect for the dignity of the guest."

It was impossible not to wonder who would do the gentle restraining should a guest go bonkers. After all, this retreat would be led by Spring Washam, a Buddhist meditation teacher from California who radiates serenity.

There were the standard admonitions about disclosing use of prescription medications, remaining sexually abstinent, and adhering to a saltless, sugarless, plant-based diet. But it was the bizarre final line

of the document that we came back to again and again as things got
weird in the days ahead.

"Finally . . . please always try to remember that Spring E. Washam
is just a simple human being trying to do her best to heal all beings
everywhere," the form concluded. "Occasionally misunderstandings
will happen. We ask for your love, compassion and forgiveness ahead
of time. Om Mani Padme Hum."

The sign-off, a Sanskrit mantra that Buddhists chant to invoke the
state of unconditional compassion, would come in handy during our
initial group meeting, when the first bombshell dropped.

We were sitting on cots inside the oval-shaped ceremony room, af-
fectionately called the Mother Ship, which was adorned with Tibetan
prayer flags and a giant quartz lamp that changed colors from neon
green to pink to blue every few seconds. Dusk was approaching as
one of Spring's deputies, Yugo Feather, a lanky Australian with im-
possibly long eyelashes, delivered a shocking piece of news matter-
of-factly. Spring, he said, would be skipping the retreat because she
was receiving medical care for a rare tropical disease.

"We will be sending her our love," he said, seeming eager to change
the subject.

I scanned the room and was met by other stunned gazes. The lore
and lure of Spring Washam was what had driven us to this remote
valley in the rainforest—but the commander of the Mother Ship had
apparently called in sick.

Many of us had read her memoir, *A Fierce Heart: Finding Strength,
Courage, and Wisdom in Any Moment*. It chronicles how Spring over-
came a turbulent life marred by sexual abuse, poverty, and a stint as a
drug dealer to become a rising star in Buddhist circles in the United
States.

We had watched her well-produced YouTube videos, in which an
unfailingly radiant and smiling Spring introduces herself as a *curan-
dera*, or traditional healer, singularly equipped to transform lives by
combining the curative power of Shipibo Indigenous ayahuasca rituals with Buddhist wisdom. "Ayahuasca is a powerful doctor, a great

healer," she said in a video posted shortly before our retreat, titled "How to Raise Your Vibration with Ayahuasca (How to Heal Negative Energy)."

In the video, Spring's teeth sparkle. Her dark olive skin glows. Her long, thick, jet-black curls are draped over her right shoulder. There is an alluring aliveness about her, a sense of otherworldly buoyancy as she hails ayahuasca's miraculous properties. It transforms our DNA by removing "traumatic imprints," she claims. It heals physical pain and autoimmune disorders that stump conventional doctors. "This powerful plant can literally help to open up our chakras and nadis to help our energy flow, thus creating balance and harmony in our bodies," she says.

These were claims long on hyperbole and short on science. But almost two years into the COVID-19 pandemic, it was tempting to give Spring the benefit of the doubt, to take her at her word. The implicit promise of her marketing is that if you follow her into the jungle and spend a couple of weeks tripping at night and listening to her dharma talks during the day, you too could reverse the aging process, slay childhood demons, and walk away looking like the epitome of health.

Yet, having paid almost $3,000 and traveled thousands of miles in defiance of pandemic-era guidance, we were told nonchalantly that the healer was too sick to tend to our ailments. Yugo was vague about Spring's condition at first, saying only that the treatment involved an intravenous drug that left her body ravaged. The show would go on without her, he assured us, and we would send her healing vibes and metta—a Buddhist term for loving-kindness—from the Mother Ship. There was no talk of refunds. Om Mani Padme Hum or bust.

〜〜 The sting of this most unwelcome revelation began easing as we went around the ceremony room introducing ourselves. The opening session of a psychedelic retreat is a bit like the pilot of a reality show. Some participants revealed only a snippet of their plotlines at first, providing vague and carefully worded justifications for having signed up for two weeks of meditating and purging under Spring's tutelage. Others spoke with striking candor, leaning on the implicit understanding that everyone who embarked on these journeys was at least a little broken.

Among them was Gary, a frail California man in his early eighties who told us he had lost the will to live after his wife had died a few years earlier. A seasoned meditator, he mentioned that he had helped organize a visit by the Dalai Lama to Los Angeles. But life had become meaningless and dull as a widower, and Gary had come to see the retreat as a final chance to extend his earthly runway.

Mike, an accountant from Australia in his late thirties, revealed that he had been in a depressive sinkhole for months. It had put his marriage on life support and made him feel inadequate and absent as a father.

I struggled to hear Lisa, a palliative care nurse, as she spoke barely above a whisper about the recent passing of her mother. I immediately liked Sonia, a talented musician with gorgeous blue eyes, who was trying to decide whether to go to graduate school or focus on her budding career as a sound healer.

Holly and Catherine, two statuesque yoga moms from the Midwest, had come to Peru together and seemed to relish the fact that they didn't tell their husbands about the nature of the retreat. There were four men who were Lotus Vine veterans.

But it was two women who were ayahuasca novices that most captured my imagination during our ice-breaking session. Tashima, a lesbian in her early seventies, was assigned a spot next to mine in the ceremony room. She revealed little in her introduction, but her blue eyes were glassy and withdrawn, seeming to hold a lot of sorrow.

Then there was Ivette, the indisputable showstopper of the retreat. When she began speaking, we all sat up a little straighter. Ivette was not her real name, she informed us, not anymore. She had been called that at birth by parents who had been emotionally and physically abusive to her and her siblings. As an adult, determined to sever all ties to them, she had legally changed her name to Fame Chanel, a rebirth of sorts that helped her to look forward rather than back as she raised children with her husband, Stanley, a retired marine. Early in the pandemic, she stumbled across an online video about ayahuasca and felt a sudden urge to resurrect Ivette, if only briefly. Stanley refused to hear any of it, but Fame got a job as a school aide in early 2020 and began saving money to go to Peru and put her inner child in Spring's care.

Speaking loudly and clearly, as though she had carefully weighed each word ahead of time, Fame told us she had decided to resurrect her birth name because she owed it to little Ivette to confront pain that had been too searing to metabolize in real time. Stanley was outraged as his normally obsequious wife had embarked on this odyssey, she said, fretting that he might be losing her to a cult. It was the first time she had acted against his will. But there was not a quiver of doubt in her voice.

〰〰 In the absence of Spring, we found consolation in the presence of Pepe Franchini Vásquez, the Shipibo maestro, or shaman, who would be leading our ceremonies. Lotus Vine hailed Pepe as one of the true masters of the Shipibo plant medicine lineage. He was the protagonist of the 2016 documentary *The Last Shaman*, which chronicles the journey of James Freeman, a suicidal young man from New England who travels to Peru in search of a genuine healer. After striking out with a series of charlatans, an emaciated and dazed Freeman finds Pepe and begins to heal under his care in Santa Rosa de Dinamarca, a riverside village in northern Peru. The documentary ends on a disquieting note as Pepe is exiled from the village for reasons that aren't explained in the film. This leaves Freeman in the lurch, like a surgery patient taken from the operating table before getting stitched up.

Pepe told me he had started his shamanic training when he was twelve years old under the guidance of an uncle, Antonio Vásquez, a preeminent Shipibo healer in the Pucallpa region. Under Antonio's supervision, he began dieting with plants and participating in ayahuasca ceremonies. The training involved long periods of sexual abstinence and seclusion, a process of withdrawal that Pepe said made it possible to merge with the world of plant spirits.

"The plants began to teach me," he said. "Just as clearly as we are speaking to each other, they say: 'Pepe, this works for this kind of sickness.'"

When I asked Pepe how he runs ceremonies, he said something that echoed what the Yawanawá had told me. Much of his energy is spent warding off curses, which Pepe described as darts set in motion by other shamans. "When it comes to medicinal plants, God created two paths: good and evil," he said. Pepe said every ailment in the soul and body has a curse at its root. During ayahuasca ceremonies, Pepe said, he scans each participant's body, trying to discern where he senses blockages. Then he sings a special song known as an *icaro*. The tunes become a form of invisible surgery that prod, push, and, when successful, ultimately dislodge bundles of darkness from the body. The Shipibo call them *malos aires*, which roughly translates to "pockets of rotten air."

〜〜 As we gathered in the Mother Ship for the first ceremony, we noticed another absence. Gary, the octogenarian from California, would be returning home the following morning, Yugo informed us, because he took a drug for a heart condition that could be dangerous with ayahuasca. How this didn't get sorted out before Gary flew four thousand miles was not addressed. We were asked to send Gary and his broken, widowed heart metta during the ceremony that night. Om Mani Padme Hum.

After the second ceremony, we lost two more participants. Holly and Catherine had experienced a terrifying bout of paranoia the evening before, Holly told me later. They had come to question the story about Spring's absence and grew convinced they had stumbled into a dangerous cult. In hushed whispers, they briefly considered running away in the middle of the night without notifying anyone. Ultimately, they cited a medical condition for their decision to abort their Lotus Vine healing journey so soon.

Ivette, meanwhile, appeared to be hanging by a thread. Her first ceremony had been terrifyingly dark, leaving her too weak and anguished to leave her room much for a couple of days. It was only days later, when she and I sat down to talk, that I grasped the monstrous trauma that had drawn her to Lotus Vine. To understand the story, it's necessary to understand that "my family are descendants from slavery," Ivette told me. The violent scourge of that history played out for generations in the form of beatings: "My mother, as a child, got beaten a lot, and her mother got beaten a lot. It was a cycle." Ivette said her mother had never shown love to her or her siblings during what she called "a terrible childhood" in an impoverished Brooklyn neighborhood.

The worst day, she said, came when she was six and Ricky, one of her siblings, was eight. He was a gentle, artistic child, and often the target of their mother's violent outbursts. "When she was beating us, she would tell us not to cry or cry out," she said. "And when we cried, she would say, 'You keep crying and I'll give you something to cry about.'" During a particularly intense beating, Ricky hollered. Their mother hit him harder. "She just kept whacking because he kept screaming and screaming and screaming," Ivette recalled. "And then he just stopped, so we felt that he just fell asleep or Mommy just stopped."

The next morning, they realized Ricky was dead. Ivette said their mother—somehow—disposed of the body. No one in the family ever brought up the subject. "Because we lived in poverty, in a ghetto situation, no one cared," Ivette said. "No one came to investigate." The scene had flashed before her eyes during the first ayahuasca ceremony. She had glimpsed the horror in her brother's eyes, saw herself cowering as her mother beat him, and took in the haunting silence that followed. The looks on everyone's faces the following day. "The whole incident just came back to me," she said. "That was the horror, that was the terror." The memory had sparked feelings of anger—toward herself. "I got mad with myself, and I wondered why I dismissed it," she said. "No one in my family talks about it. No one talks about Ricky. Like he didn't exist, but he did exist."

〰〰 Halfway through the retreat, we went on a hike to a waterfall near the lodge and I found myself walking alongside Tashima, my seatmate on the Mother Ship. I admired her meditation posture and the ease she projected, even though it was hard to tell whether it reflected a state of calm or resignation. We were discussing mundane things on the hilly trail, like how she wound up living in New Mexico and how long she had been meditating, when Tashima told me, as naturally as someone might say they're ready to quit their job, that she had decided she would end her life soon. It was time to finally surrender to a thought that had lurked in her mind with varying degrees of intensity for much of her life. "I sort of feel like I just don't belong here," she said.

Tashima said that earlier in life she had been an activist, passionate about the power of ordinary people to shift the course of history for the better. She walked across the United States in 1986 as part of the Great Peace March, calling for nuclear disarmament. Wanderlust kept her motivated over the years: she spent weeks hiking through the Himalayas and walked to Machu Picchu. About a decade earlier, Tashima said, she became embroiled in a tragedy. A teenage boy who participated in a white water rafting excursion run by a program she managed got trapped underwater for several minutes and became severely disabled. The boy's parents sued the program and directed their wrath toward Tashima. They brought the wheelchair-bound boy to her deposition, an image that unsettled her then and haunts her now.

In recent years, as her body grew frail and the world more frenetic, Tashima told me, she had run out of reasons to stay alive. She was childless, single, and had meager earnings. And the election of Donald Trump in 2016 exacerbated her sense of dread. "It felt hopeless," she said. "It's like, where is this world going? Where is this country going?"

We walked the last stretch of the hike in silence. I was haunted by what Tashima had just shared and shaken by the brutal scene Ivette had described earlier. I realized then that, beyond the body-convulsing tripping and the lure of the ritual, there's a simple and perhaps paramount reason these retreats can be so healing. In these settings, we get to take on the pain of others, to share the burden of losses, big and small, of the regrets and the split-second horrors that diverted a person's destiny. With that comes a realization that we are less alone than we presumed, less likely to be stigmatized than we feared, less atypical in our ambivalence about staying alive. If I had crossed paths with Ivette or Tashima as seatmates on a long flight, I would have looked away, made quick assumptions about them. And I would have walked away poorer for not knowing a bit about their sorrow, the memories that kept them up at night, the events that turned their hair gray and their eyes doleful.

〰〰 The night after that conversation with Tashima, I spent much of the first half of the ceremony standing on the deck of the Mother Ship, gazing at the stars. Pepe's *icaros* had grown intolerable, so before heading down to the maloca, I had grabbed some contraband: my phone, which had been on airplane mode during the retreat, and a pair of earbuds. Standing in a dark spot, I stuck one in each ear and scrolled through my playlists looking for one I had created six months earlier, shortly after impulsively saying "I love you" to a man I had known for less than a week. Titled "Trust the System," it was a compilation of thirty-two songs that spoke to the mysterious and vertigo-inducing process of falling in love.

The months before meeting Steve, the recipient of the playlist, were among the hardest of my life. In the fall of 2020, I traveled to Colombia to tend to my father, who was being obliterated by cancer.

During his final weeks, he became incontinent and deranged as purple tumors disfigured his neck and forehead. He asked strange, dark questions, like whether I knew that Ernest Hemingway had ended his life with a self-inflicted bullet. I asked whether he was considering suicide. He smiled mischievously and let the question drown in the awful silence that followed. One afternoon, as we sat next to each other on his terrace, I gently suggested that there might be something to look forward to in whatever happens after death. He cut me short, making clear he didn't believe anything transcends the end of a beating heart. Yet, on his final, restless night, my father did something that suggests he may have had a change of heart: he began crying and reaching out from bed as he called out, "Natalia, Natalia, Natalia!" Had morphine made him hallucinate the spirit of his mother, pulling him toward whatever comes next? Or—my grieving mind reeled—is it possible that our ancestors are capable of reaching into this earthly domain at crucial moments—to protect us from harm, to steer us, and perhaps to draw us back to them?

In the months following his death, under the crush of walloping grief, I took solace in the latter possibility and allowed it to unspool wildly in my mind. Grief gave me a license to suspend disbelief, to entertain paranormal beliefs, to dabble in prayer, realizing how starved I had been for faith. The low point came in January 2021, when, back in Rio de Janeiro and trying to turn my mind back to work, I developed a severe case of COVID-19 and had to be hospitalized for nearly a week. Gasping for air and feeling utterly alone in an intensive care room, I turned to prayer. I prayed to my father, asking him to send me a good man, a partner, someone who would help me go through life feeling less alone.

As someone who was trying faith on for size, I added a special request: this man should be wearing something red when I met him, a feature rare enough it would convince me when I saw him that he had indeed been heaven-sent.

A few months later, scrolling on a dating app on a Friday night, I saw the profile of a handsome man visiting from Minnesota for the weekend. He was a vegetarian and a veterinarian. Swoon. And free health care for Hugo to boot!

I invited him to go on a bike ride the next day. He accepted. The next morning, I walked out to greet him, secretly looking for a loud red T-shirt. Alas, it was gray, with a logo that had minuscule dashes of a red-adjacent hue. Close enough? After the bike ride, we went to a beach and then to dinner, and by nighttime, it was clear that he would spend the night.

The next day, Steve asked if I would consider tagging along for his remaining week in Brazil, which included visits to an island and a small colonial town. There was nothing terribly pressing on my agenda; I took the week off. The night before his trip home, lying in bed in the dark, I told Steve, "I love you," words I had become wary of uttering, especially early in a relationship. He said he loved me too. We both seemed to understand we had stumbled into something precious, by divine intervention or dumb luck, and that we were going to give it a whirl.

Within a couple of weeks, Steve was back in Rio. During the pandemic, much of his job as a university professor could be done remotely, so he began spending far more time in Brazil than in Minnesota. Living together was a breeze, and we made each other laugh a lot. By the time I went to Lotus Vine, we hadn't figured out what a future together might look like, what career sacrifices it might entail or whether the honeymoon stage of our courtship would lead to a lasting, deep bond. But that night, listening to the songs in that playlist, in flagrant violation of Mother Ship rules, I decided there was no doubt that my heartfelt prayer had been answered. I listened to two of the songs we liked most in that list: "Bless the Broken Road," by Rascal Flatts, and a Mexican ranchera that has always given me goose bumps, "Si Nos Dejan"—"If They Let Us." Each note seemed to push me to expand my capacity for love a bit more, to trust that this could work, to realize that *this* was what I would prioritize, because it was suddenly so clear that nothing mattered more than love.

It must have been well past midnight when I went back inside, asked for a second serving of ayahuasca, and lay back on my mat. When the ceremony ended, Tashima reached out and asked if she could hug me. I had no memory of it, but she told me I had cried for what seemed like hours after coming back inside, at times gently, at times sobbing. She wrapped her bony arms around me and said words that make me tear up every time I remember them: "You are so worthy of love."

〰 With Spring's dharma talks canceled, the most Buddhist-adjacent offerings of the retreat were yoga classes taught by a comically chirpy Canadian woman called Acacia. She had moved to Tarapoto, in Peru, a few years earlier to live with her husband, a Peruvian musician and *ayahuasquero*. In addition to teaching yoga almost every day of the retreat, and at Spring's request, Acacia gave us a lecture on how to integrate the insights and lessons of the retreat in our daily lives.

Her slow vinyasa yoga classes, set to soothing new age music, were designed to make our bodies and minds more receptive to "the medicine," a term she rattled off every other chaturanga. "You are in a very safe container, where you can continue to go deeper and deeper in your process," she said during a morning practice. "When you feel things start to come up within yourself, have the courage to surrender and allow yourself to go fully into your process, because that's where the medicine has the power to cure."

Her quirkiness notwithstanding, I took a liking to Acacia and overlooked a couple of shocking word choices she used to guide us into poses. She referred to the pose commonly known as "happy baby"—lying on your back while holding your feet with your hands, legs spread apart—as "happy husband." One day, she instructed us to contort our legs in the shape of a "swastika"—a prompt that elicited muffled gasps. But it was during one of her final classes that she made the comment that would get her fired from Lotus Vine and spark a reckoning that thrust Spring into damage control mode. Acacia mentioned that she and her husband also ran ayahuasca retreats at a nearby center and that they would be happy to host us there in the future. I asked her what the name of the center was and felt my body jolt when she responded. "Katari," she said. I wondered if I had misheard, so I followed up, asking her what her husband's name was. "Herbert Quintero," she replied. I had heard correctly.

Katari and Herbert Quintero had become radioactive in ayahuasca social media circles after a woman named Sina posted a video on Facebook in March 2021 describing sexual harassment she experienced after a retreat she attended in Peru. After rolling up my mat, I went to my room and looked up the video to jog my memory about the nature of the allegations.

In the thirteen-minute video, Sina said that after she left the retreat, Herbert incessantly sent her flirtatious messages, which she displayed in the video, firing off one after another: "Miss you; Feeling u my love; Love u; Wanna be there with you; Miss u."

Sina said she sometimes turned to Herbert when she was feeling particularly depressed, because she had come to see him as a healer. During a video call one day, she said, he asked her if she masturbated regularly. "He asked me if I would masturbate for him on camera because it would open up my sacral chakra and it would help me heal," she recounted tearfully in the video. "And I'm very embarrassed to admit that I did, because I was looking for healing and I trusted him. I trusted him a lot."

Sina said she was too embarrassed to tell anyone for a long time, but when she finally broke down and told a friend, the friend said she had experienced a similar interaction with Herbert when she was emotionally vulnerable. After the video was posted in an ayahuasca group on Facebook with thousands of users, a deluge of similar allegations poured in. Some said Herbert had sexually assaulted them after ceremonies. This is far from the first sex-abuse scandal I had followed in the psychedelics world. But one thing stood out: the damage control strategy. Soon after Sina's video was posted, Katari's Facebook account posted a statement attributed to "Herbert's wife." It was Acacia, our yoga instructor. And her response was by turns revelatory, obfuscating, and gaslighting. "What he did was wrong and he made a mistake," Acacia wrote. "We don't need to condemn him or label him as a predator because that is not what he is." What he is, she added, is someone with "boundary issues, and although this was new to the public, we have been working to heal this together for a long time."

She added that Herbert had stepped down as director of his retreat and urged anyone else "who has been hurt" to leave a comment on the post. Acacia also made a case for her husband's comeback: "Herbert's thing to work on is filling the hole he has within himself that kept him seeking love and acknowledgement from the outside," she said. "He is talented at holding groups within medicine journeys and it would be a shame for him to walk away from this all together [sic]."

A nagging question kept me up that night: Did Spring know that she had hired the wife and business partner of a man accused of sexual harassment and assault?

Spring promoted her retreat as the safest in the business. She also spent a lot of time on social media, where the accusations against Herbert, and Acacia's justification of his behavior, were easy to find in the small world of ayahuasca retreats. And yet she had hired Acacia, who was now recruiting people at Lotus Vine.

This question about Spring led to a personal one: Did I have a responsibility to speak out? I decided I did and raised the issue publicly during our next group meeting. When I finished speaking, Yugo looked mortified. He said he and Spring had long known who Herbert was and the accusations against him. Jaws dropped. A few hours later, we were summoned to a meeting in the Mother Ship. And as we approached, we heard a singsongy voice we recognized from the You-Tube videos. A convalescent Spring had come to address the question on everyone's mind: What on earth was she thinking?

Spring told us she had met Acacia after seeing a flyer for yoga lessons in Tarapoto. They clicked when Acacia came for an interview, but at the end of the conversation, when Acacia mentioned in passing who her husband was, Spring said she was horrified and deemed the relationship a deal-breaker. But Acacia begged for the job, she said, saying the couple was broke and that Herbert had nearly died from COVID and was no longer running retreats. Spring said she convinced herself that hiring Acacia was a means to help her break free from a misguided marriage.

"I got this idea that I could heal her," she said. Then Spring looked inward and said she was shaken by her lapse in judgment. "I hope we can find a lesson, a higher teacher, that will make my energy around Lotus Vine more protective."

〰 The day after our sixth and final ceremony at Lotus Vine, we gathered in the Mother Ship one last time to share our impressions. Tashima said her heart had been blasted open during the final ceremony, filling her with incandescent love. Then and there, she decided she had one more major hike to cross off her list before checking out from life: she intended to walk the five-hundred-mile Camino de Santiago, in Spain. Her savings were limited, and, at seventy, it would be a challenge. But suddenly, being alive felt like a precious gift. And this bold plan made her feel something she hadn't felt in a long time, she said: excited, resolute, joyful.

Then Ivette spoke to report a startling breakthrough. During her last ceremony, as she descended into a spiral of nausea and despair, a familiar face emerged. Her mother, who died years earlier from breast cancer, appeared and leaned in for a hug. "She embraced me, and she was full of light and love," Ivette said, tears streaming down her cheeks. "She kept saying, 'I'm so proud of you. You did good.'" It was her first taste of motherly love, Ivette said. That vision, whether real or imagined, shifted something profound within her. "I felt the love, and I felt I was complete," Ivette said.

〰 A few weeks after we left Peru, Spring sent an email to people who had booked upcoming retreats. Another shoe was about to drop. Lotus Vine was ceasing operations in the country, she announced, and the retreat that followed ours was the last to feature Shipibo healers.

"Due to some very serious ethical issues that arose during our November 2021 retreat, we have ceased all communication and work with Pepe Vasquez Franchini," Spring wrote, calling it "heartbreaking." He was the fifth Peruvian ayahuasca maestro she had fired, Spring went on.

This was a shocking development. The Shipibo system had been a central feature of Spring's retreats; now she seemed to be shifting responsibility for any problems with her operation onto the Indigenous healers and cutting them out.

And what happened to Pepe? To get his side of the story, I reached him in Spain, where he was leading ceremonies at retreats run by Russians.

Pepe told me that toward the end of the retreat that followed ours, Spring and her assistants had summoned him to a meeting and told him they had learned that he had once fondled a young woman in his village, and told him to leave. The accusation was not true, Pepe said, but he didn't see a point in pushing back. "I didn't make a fuss," he told me.

But leaving Peru, and the Shipibo tradition, behind did not mean Spring was getting out of the ayahuasca business. Her operation moved to Costa Rica, where her focus shifted. Instead of catering to run-of-the-mill suffering souls, Lotus Vine Journeys, Costa Rica edition, would cater to people on a mission. The updated marketing material called on "teachers, thought leaders and activists" who "dream of creating a better world and are already creating it" to book their spot. Turbocharging those dreams would not be cheap: the Costa Rica journeys cost $7,480, more than twice what we paid in Peru. No Shipibo healers would be on hand, but Spring's new retreats would be infused with teachings of the life of the American abolitionist Harriet Tubman, the subject of her new book.

I followed the plot twists at Lotus Vine with bewilderment and fascination, trading notes often with a handful of retreat participants who became close friends. On closer inspection, there was something jarringly improvisational about Spring's operation. One day, Shipibo healers were central to her healing marathon. The next, they were expendable—shifty figures who simply could not be trusted.

And what were we to make of Pepe, who had convinced all of us that he had real mastery of his craft, eliciting visceral sensations—and vomit—with his songs? Was he a mild-mannered predator in a field in which sexual abuse often gets swept under the rug? Or had he simply been caught up in shamanic bad blood?

One thing became clear in the months ahead: Spring was hardly an aberration in the psychedelics retreat field. To a large extent, it has been shaped by wounded people who stumbled into psychedelics during a dark night of the soul and emerged with a messianic complex. I've heard many say they received an unmistakable message from the spiritual realm during a powerful ceremony that led them to believe they had been tapped as force multipliers in a world in dire need of healing. Those who step into such roles and build successful franchises tend to have confidence in spades, a knack for marketing, and a willingness to take enormous risks.

Despite my personal breakthroughs and those I had watched on retreats, it soon became clear to me that when you're administering psychoactive drugs to people in distress, a lot can go terribly wrong. Given the murky legality of the trade—in which hold-harmless agreements are the norm—when people are seriously hurt, there's often little recourse. That became painfully clear to a handful of women who arrived in Peru soon after the end of our retreat, for an adventure that quickly turned into a nightmare.

7   A RAPE IN THE RAINFOREST

MICHELLE SÁNCHEZ MET THE MAN who would soon rape her at a restaurant called Karma Café. She was among a group of eight women who traveled thousands of miles to the Peruvian city of Iquitos in early November 2021 to learn from one of the masters of a jungle healing modality known as kambo. The curative arsenal of native communities in the Amazon includes several tough-love medicines. But kambo is in a league of its own. The elixir is extracted by subjecting giant leaf frogs to stress, often by strapping them onto a small cross and dangling their slimy bodies near an open flame. The stress makes the amphibians secrete a toxic milky goo. To administer it, kambo practitioners make a handful of burn wounds on a patient's bicep or leg and dab a bit of the frog's discharge on the raw skin.

Kambo, a frog venom rich in bioactive peptides, jolts the nervous system into an anaphylaxis-like state within seconds. Often it makes the heart thump like a manic drum. The face and limbs swell like balloons. Nausea builds up in a crescendo until the stomach revolts with bouts of green-and-pink projectile vomit. As the sting wears off, kambo patients say they experience an astounding sense of ease, as though the body has just undergone a hard reset. To call the buildup unpleasant is an understatement: kambo would be an effective form of torture. But many people who have hit rock bottom and found little reprieve in allopathic medicine have come to see kambo as a Hail Mary, in some cases a literal lifesaver.

Those were the sort of people drawn to Kambo Jungle Expeditions, whose founder, Victor Escobar, promised not only to treat visitors with the potent frog medicine but to train them to administer it themselves. His website, featuring a photo of Victor with a massive anaconda draped over his shoulders, claims that kambo can treat everything from infertility to Parkinson's disease, Alzheimer's disease, depression, cancer, and heart attacks.

"The advice I give to people who have terminal illness, PLEASE don't feel bad and TRUST IN NATURE," Victor wrote on the website. "Kambo can help you in everything."

Michelle didn't need much convincing. She spent much of her childhood and adolescence in a web of depression.

"Starting around eleven years old, I started to become really depressed and experienced a lot of suicidal ideation and self-harming in the form of cutting or burning myself," she told me. She first tried this Indigenous ritual that leaves lasting burn scars years ago; it was her saving grace, she said.

Kambo was a treatment of last resort for Tabatha Marie Hammer, a fellow retreat participant. A victim of sexual trafficking who told me she was abused from the age of twelve until her midtwenties, Tabatha had tried every conventional treatment known as she struggled with post-traumatic stress, addiction, and homelessness. After watching a documentary about kambo, she felt that she had nothing to lose. "Even if I poisoned myself and died, it wouldn't really matter," she explained. "At least I was trying to help myself."

Tabatha, who became a kambo practitioner, saw the trip to the Amazon as a rare opportunity to hone her skills in the birthplace of the healing ritual, where she would get to treat local villagers. "It's kind of an honor that you would be able to serve people in the Amazon," she told me.

Kailey Horsley, a third retreat participant, had also found so much healing for her depression in kambo that she too began administering what she came to call a "warrior medicine."

The journey from Utah to Iquitos was her first trip abroad. Kailey recalled being terrified until she set foot inside a back room of Karma Café, which was decorated with psychedelic art and colorful lamps strung from the ceiling. Inside were Victor, who had a mop of jet-black curly hair, and his partner, Natasha, a Canadian kambo practitioner, and their two toddlers. Over dinner, Victor and Natasha told the retreat participants that Natasha would be staying behind to take care of the kids. It was disappointing news, several women told me, but it made sense.

"He was super charismatic and super nice," Kailey said. "Once I met him, I was like, 'I made it. I'm safe, with people I can trust.'"

〰〰 It's easy to miss, but if you read the Kambo Jungle Expeditions website closely, you'll find two versions of Victor's origin story—with a striking discrepancy. One says he was born in Iquitos in 1986, in a small village in the jungle, where he was raised by his parents. Click on another tab, and you'll read that Victor was actually born in Brazil near the Amazon River. There, he writes, he learned about "a magical medicine called Kambo" from the Katukina tribe. For years, he administered kambo to himself and others, which Victor said helped him grow spiritually, physically, mentally, and emotionally. "I helped a lot of people with their ailments and diseases and I found profound happiness in helping them," he wrote.

Starting in 2017, he and Natasha began hosting seven-night retreats at a riverside center near the forest that consists of a cluster of simple wooden buildings decorated with murals that pay homage to the kambo frog, Indigenous elders, and jaguars. One room is decorated with the skulls of two black caimans, one of the biggest predators of the Amazon.

Ayahuasca ceremonies were a core offering of Victor's retreat, but the main draw was learning how to gather, prepare, and administer kambo. Participants are urged to approach retreats as a pilgrimage of sorts, an opportunity to connect with the essence of kambo and seek its permission to amplify its healing powers. "You should go directly to this magical creature and ask permission, give your thanks, and connect one on one," Victor's website instructs.

Michelle found that idea deeply resonant. A fluent Spanish speaker with an insatiable thirst for knowledge about the traditional medicines of the Amazon, she found herself peppering Victor with questions.

"I'm very big on receiving teachings," she told me. So she was riveted by Victor's tales of kambo and his reverence for the frog. During the first full day of the retreat, a Monday, when the women went deep into the jungle to collect the medicine, she said Victor began showering her with compliments. Their friendly banter led Victor to start making lustful comments, she said. Michelle initially wondered if her natural warmth had been misinterpreted. "I know I wasn't being flirtatious," she told me almost a year after the retreat. "I was just being an openhearted person."

At first, she opted to shrug it off and give him the benefit of the doubt. But then Victor began whispering, "*Me gustas*," or "I like you," and lamenting that he was having little sex with Natasha. Later that day, Michelle sought to put an end to Victor's overtures, shutting him down politely but firmly. "I don't feel the same way," she recalled telling him. "I want you to know that I see you as a teacher, as a friend, and nothing else." For good measure, she added, "I don't want anything to happen between us."

They had their first nighttime ayahuasca ceremony. Michelle felt confident that she had established a clear boundary and set out to soak in all the lessons the retreat stood to offer.

At night, she and a couple of the other guests sat in the darkened maloca as Victor held court, telling them frightening stories about the spirits of the jungle. There was a downpour, and the darkness inside the ceremony room was briefly interrupted by bolts of lightning.

The women were sleep-deprived and still slightly buzzed from the ayahuasca ceremony the night before. Victor served them two other Indigenous medicines: sananga, eye drops derived from Mata Heins root, which sting powerfully when administered, but are said to enhance a person's eyesight and focus; and rapé, a dried, powdered tobacco that is blown into a person's nostrils using a V-shaped tube. As midnight approached, two of the women went to bed. Michelle wanted to join them, but Victor asked her to stay.

"I want to talk to you," he pleaded. "I am really enjoying this space." Michelle agonized over her decision in the minutes that followed. She wanted to leave, she told me, but heeded Victor's request. Soon, Michelle said, Victor began kissing and fondling her. She realizes she could have screamed, shoved him aside, and put an end to Victor's unwanted advances. But instead, she told me, she resisted—gently, quietly. "I don't feel the same," she remembers telling him. "I don't want to do this." But Victor pressed on, and soon he was penetrating her, Michelle recalled.

"During the act, at some point, I built the courage to say, 'Please stop—I don't want to do this,'" she told me. Victor pressed on for a while but soon pulled out, she said. Then he began pleading once more, telling Michelle that he had primal needs his wife wasn't meeting. Then he flattered her effusively, telling Michelle she was "so powerful, a strong medicine woman," she said.

When it was over, Michelle quietly made her way to the tiny room she shared with Kailey. She felt stunned, and agonized over whether she could have prevented the assault.

Did Victor's actions amount to rape? It was a question that tormented her that night and continued to haunt her in the months ahead. Sure, she could have screamed, but doing so could have brought the retreat to a sudden halt. Michelle was certain she had not consented to having sex with Victor. Was consent even possible in a setting where everyone is consuming mind-altering substances?

Perhaps she had a duty to tell the other women what happened the next morning, Michelle recalls thinking. But she didn't. "I didn't want to ruin anyone's time," she explained. "One woman had come from Europe. She had traveled so far." Michelle said she worried she may have inadvertently led Victor on. "I was kind of blaming myself," she said. "Maybe I shouldn't have been as nice."

〰〰 The following day, Michelle had a major breakdown after being administered kambo. "I have never cried so much sitting with kambo," she told me. "I felt so much in my heart, so much heaviness and grief and pain just coming out of me, and I knew where it came from, I knew I didn't have it before." She yearned to confide in someone about the assault, but words failed her. The closest she got was asking Kailey a vague question: "Have you ever been in a situation in which you did something you didn't want to do?" Their exchange didn't progress from generalities. Kailey would only make sense of Michelle's question the following day.

That night, the eight women huddled inside the maloca for the second ayahuasca ceremony of the retreat. Victor sat on mats set in the center of the ceremony room alongside Sara Ramírez, a Shipibo Indigenous maestra who sang *icaros* with her son. Kailey's first ayahuasca ceremony had been terrifying, so she brought the cup to her lips with trepidation. But she experienced bliss that night, she said. When Sara announced the ceremony had come to a close, Kailey remained on her mat, feeling radiant and too dizzy to stand.

Victor tiptoed toward her in the dark and asked Kailey in a whisper if she would blow some rapé into his nose. She would be delighted, Kailey recalled telling him. Victor began rubbing the soles of her feet with copaiba oil, telling Kailey it would help her "get back into your body." It was unexpected, she said, but Kailey assumed it was merely a friendly gesture. "We were having a great conversation," she recalled. "He is so charismatic and has a way of making it seem completely innocent to the point where you think you might be overreacting." Victor told Kailey that he saw enormous potential in her, and was sure she would become a "great medicine woman," she said. He offered her free kambo to take home and told her she was welcome to come back on another retreat for free because they were now friends. "It felt amazing because he was a well-known, well-respected teacher in the community saying that he believes in me and believes that I'm going to help a lot of people," Kailey said.

But soon things got creepy. Victor told Kailey she should move to Iquitos and offered to help her find land in the jungle, where she could run retreats of her own. His hands began slithering up her leg, Kailey said. Seeking to shut him down gently, Kailey brought up Natasha, which prompted Victor once again to unload about his marriage. "We're in a weird place," Kailey remembers him saying. "I don't know if it's going to work out." Kailey told him in no uncertain terms that she was happily married. "I was trying my best to not blatantly be like, 'Stop touching me,'" she said. "I wanted to give him the benefit of the doubt." Victor hardened the grip on her legs and kept moving his hands upward, she told me, prompting Kailey to say, "I don't want anything more than friendship with you." He pressed on, she said. "I was honestly terrified," Kailey said. "I was pulling his hands off me, but he was stronger, and there was nothing I could do."

Daylight was her salvation. As dawn broke, they heard the kitchen staff walking around the maloca. That gave Kailey an opening to press her body off the ground and return to her room.

Locking eyes with Michelle, Kailey asked, "Hey, has Victor been creepy toward you?"

Michelle's heart sank.

"What did he do to you?" Michelle asked.

After exchanging stories, they were startled. Michelle and Kailey decided they needed to tell the other retreat participants, but quietly, while they figured out an exit strategy. It suddenly dawned on them just how reliant they were on Victor.

"We had no idea how to get back to Iquitos," Kailey said. "We were completely relying on him for our safety, to get out of the jungle— everything." The center had no internet connection and no cell phone service. After Kailey and Michelle broke the news to the rest of the group during breakfast, the other women were outraged. A third participant disclosed that during the first ayahuasca ceremony, Victor had rubbed copaiba oil on her feet after the ceremony and called her a "strong medicine woman" as he fondled her legs. The fondling stopped when another participant summoned Victor.

〰 Kailey and Michelle decided to pull Maestra Sara aside. If someone was in a position to help and protect them, it was this medicine woman in her late fifties, they figured. With Michelle translating, the women told Sara what Victor had done. "At first, she thought we were having visions of Victor touching us and talked about how the medicine can sometimes bring different visions," Kailey said. The women said they were certain they hadn't collectively hallucinated Victor's problematic behavior. Sara then said something that left them speechless. "We all hold a lot of dark energy," Michelle recalled Sara saying. "He's still working on a lot."

Seeing how upset the women were, Sara promised that she would protect them during the final days of the retreat—but she also encouraged them to let bygones be bygones.

"This is what happens in women's lives sometimes, and we just have to deal with it, accept it, and move on," the maestra said. The women left the meeting baffled.

It didn't take long for Victor to pick up on the palpable sense of anxiety that had taken hold among his guests. Tabatha and another participant, an army veteran named Lisa, confronted Victor about his actions and demanded to be taken back to Iquitos at once.

"Pure panic set in," said Tabatha, noting that several women had turned to kambo partly to heal from sexual trauma. "You had all these girls in fight-or-flight mode and it all became a little insane."

Victor initially denied the allegations. Then he said the women may have misinterpreted his actions. Ultimately, he broke down in tears and asked for forgiveness, at one point getting on his knees, Kailey, Michelle, and Tabatha told me in separate interviews. He told them his was a lonely line of work and that he struggled to contain his sexual impulses. "I haven't had people offer me guidance to further my healing," Michelle remembers him saying. "It's just me out here."

Victor said it was impossible to arrange for a boat ride to Iquitos sooner than the scheduled departure date, which was two nights away. He pleaded with them to take advantage of their remaining time in the jungle and said he still had so much to show and teach them. But the women balked. That day, they all crammed into two of the rooms far from Victor's, assuming they would be safer if they stuck together. A couple considered stealing one of the boats at the center, but they had no idea how they would operate it or what direction to take. Fearing Victor might assault them again, the women armed themselves with knives from the kitchen and bat-size sticks from the forest. "We didn't sleep the rest of the time," Tabatha said.

Victor spent the final days of the retreat locked up in his room, saying he was feeling ill. The day of their departure, Sara summoned the women for a farewell meeting. She presented them with gifts—traditional necklaces and tapestries from Shipibo artisans—and asked how everyone was feeling. The gesture was met with icy glares. Sara said she wanted the women to be certain that "she would make sure that Victor would not hurt any more women," Kailey told me. "You girls are like my children, and I want you to know I will protect women here."

Then Sara urged the girls not to speak about what they experienced when they returned home, arguing that livelihoods were at stake. Sitting next to her was her granddaughter. "She was telling us that with this money she was able to support her granddaughter, support her family," Michelle recalled.

Peru's economy was one of the hardest hit in the region by the COVID-19 pandemic. The United Nations in 2022 reported that more than sixteen million Peruvians experienced food insecurity—a crisis on stark display in the streets of Iquitos, where barefoot children begged tourists for change and scraps of food. The women understood that if they ratted Victor out, there was a good chance Sara would lose her job, and families in nearby villages who relied on income from the center would go hungry. "It felt like she was trying to bribe us, silence us, kind of guilt us," Michelle told me.

〰 By the time they boarded the boat to return to Iquitos on the morning of November 13, the women were exhausted. Victor spent the ride in silence, holding his face in his hands much of the three-hour journey, they said. Back in Iquitos, the women checked into a hotel and sent a message to Natasha, Victor's partner, summoning her for a meeting. Natasha met them at the DoubleTree Hilton hotel, where they told her what had happened. Natasha, who wrote on her website that Victor introduced her to kambo in 2017, appeared shocked and apologized profusely, the women said. She offered to reimburse the $1,500 each participant paid and assured them the center would close.

"She cried a little bit and was just like, 'I can't believe that I'm hearing this,'" Kailey recalled. Kailey debated whether to go public about what had happened. Doing so would not be without risk. Would she want prospective employers to know she had traveled to Peru to take a mind-altering brew and a medicine made from toxic frog secretions? Would people blame her and her fellow participants for putting themselves in such a vulnerable position? And would taking down a revered figure in the kambo world make her a pariah in a field she was passionate about? But she would do it, she said.

"When I thought about the potential impact this could have on me versus the potential impact on however many women might go there in the future, it wasn't even a question," Kailey told me.

Soon after arriving in the United States, she posted a video on Facebook recounting the events at the retreat, calling them a "nightmarish experience." Kailey's account was strikingly detailed and her rendering composed. "He knows people look up to him," she said, "and uses that to manipulate women."

Messages poured into Kailey's Facebook inbox. Scores of women told her they had been sexually assaulted or harassed by Victor. One woman wrote to Kailey that Victor raped her in September 2019 during a retreat. "He came into my hut and pushed me on a bed, touched me inappropriately," she wrote, according to screen grabs Kailey shared with me. "He penetrated me. I said NO but he wouldn't stop. I remember thunder and rain started in the jungle. I resisted. He was too strong to fight with him. He left me on the bed after he was done. I had a full on panic attack."

Another wrote: "Thank you for your video Sister. I was there almost exactly a year ago and also experienced things that I should have spoke up about. Have much regret about it." Kailey compiled the testimonies she received into a database that had more than thirty names.

In the days that followed, Natasha told the retreat participants that she had gotten to the bottom of Victor's deplorable behavior. The culprit, she informed them, was Sara, the Shipibo maestra. Natasha explained that during the retreat, Sara had prescribed Victor a diet of piñón colorado, one of the master plants in the Shipibo tradition used to connect with powerful spirits. "I still don't feel like any of what happened is OK," Natasha wrote, according to screen grabs of her messages, which Kailey shared with me. Victor, Natasha added, should never have been on a powerful plant diet while hosting a retreat. The women had experienced a deluded version of Victor, she said, and assured them that he was getting the help he needed. "He was not himself," Natasha wrote. "Tomorrow we go to someone who hopefully can help."

〰️ Daniela Peluso, an anthropologist who has studied sexual abuse in shamanic retreats in the Amazon, wrote in a 2014 article that sexual abuse of women who go to the jungle for healing has become commonplace. Foreigners drawn to the jungle to experience Indigenous rituals in their birthplace often romanticize shamans and local healers, who in turn frequently have misguided assumptions about women who come from abroad, Dr. Peluso wrote. In Peru, "there is a predominant notion that, in most circumstances, women will surrender to male sexual advances if they find themselves in a vulnerable position or merely alone with a man, as such behavior is aligned with gender expectations," she wrote. "In most contexts, any time men and women are together, there is a constant barrage of sexual overtones that inform all verbal and nonverbal behavior. To circumvent vulnerability, Indigenous women avoid smiling directly at men, laughing with them, paying too much attention to them, being in their presence without close kin nearby, and traveling alone."

As it turns out, Victor had been accused of rape before. In 2010, a young woman from California told the police in Iquitos that Victor, who was then working as a guide at a company called Amazon Adventure Expedition, raped her in a hotel room. The woman said she fended him off by spraying Mace on his face. Victor was locked up briefly, but a judge soon let him out, citing a lack of evidence in the case, according to a local press report.

In the days after leaving the jungle, Tabatha and Kailey said they wondered why it took so long for women to speak up about Victor's conduct.

"I think he's a very skilled groomer," said Tabatha, who told me that having been sexually abused as a teenager gave her an understanding into how victims often come to rationalize and excuse predatory conduct. "He knows how to get in their head." Women who have found healing in shamanic rituals that use psychedelics are often afraid of taking on well-respected figures, Tabatha said. "To come out and say something about somebody who is on a pedestal, you don't want to be that person that steps up first and says this might have happened," she said.

After having extensive conversations with Kailey, Tabatha, and Michelle and finding their accounts were consistent, I wanted to interview Sara, the maestra, as well as Natasha and Victor. They would help me fully understand what happened.

When I got her on the phone, the maestra was warm and forthcoming. She told me she had learned to lead ayahuasca ceremonies from her grandparents a little over a decade earlier. Since then, she had worked at several foreigner-run retreat centers near Iquitos, catering mainly to tourists who came with "bad energies," including many "*drogados*," or drug addicts.

The tone of her voice changed when I mentioned Victor Escobar. After a sigh, she told me, "I didn't witness anything." Based on conversations with the retreat participants, Sara told me she had come to conclude that Victor had "*manoseado*," or fondled, a few while he was "*mareado*," or dizzy from the effects of ayahuasca. Sara described the transgressions as relatively minor and said that Victor appeared to be mortified when she spoke to him the day after the second ayahuasca ceremony.

Sara said Victor was anguished about how Natasha would react if the women spoke up and pleaded with her to calm them down. "He got down on his knees and began crying," Sara told me. Sara said Victor told her, "I made a mistake. Please help me."

She gave Victor a stern talking-to. "Behave from now on," she recalled telling him, "if you want to continue working with foreigners."

Later that day, when she met with the women, Sara said she tried to comfort them and turn Victor's transgressions into a teachable moment. "It's a mistake, and everybody makes mistakes," she recalled telling them. "These are experiences we are gaining as women."

Victor and Natasha, who was born in Canada, list their cell phone numbers on their websites. Seconds after I sent Natasha a text message identifying myself as a journalist interested in speaking to her about the November 2021 retreat, my phone rang. Natasha told me that she and Victor had been eager to break their silence about what happened during the retreat. "There's a lot of lies," she told me. In essence, she told me that after Kailey posted her video, several women who had sex with Victor during retreats came to reframe their experiences and change their minds about whether the acts were consensual. "Now it becomes a thing that someone else did and they had no part in it," Natasha told me.

I mentioned the 2010 rape arrest and the dozens of accounts that Kailey had collected.

"I see him as an unhealed person who is now trying to do his work," she said.

Natasha said Victor should not have been running retreats, which she said can be hotbeds of "sexual energy," but that as far as she was concerned, his only sin was infidelity.

I pointed out how vulnerable psychedelic retreat participants can be when they're sleep-deprived and under the influence of powerful mind-altering drugs, and asked if sex that happens between a teacher and a student in that setting can ever be construed as consensual.

"I think he absolutely took advantage as far as his relationship of him being a teacher and student," she allowed. But she told me Victor never saw it that way. "I think he was just, like, happy to be there and happy to be around all these women, trying his luck."

About twelve minutes into our call, Natasha said it was Victor who should be answering questions about his behavior. After we hung up, I sat in stunned silence, trying to make sense of her steadfast support for Victor.

I needed to hear from Victor directly. I sent him a text message, and within seconds, his name was on my caller ID. He sounded anguished and unleashed a torrent of words before I could formulate an opening question.

"These women, honestly, completely destroyed my name," Victor said. "I shut down my company, my name has been dragged through the mud, and no one has listened to my version."

I was all ears. Victor told me that he had often seduced female retreat participants but that he never forced himself on anyone or fondled women who were impaired by ayahuasca. "I flirted, bantered, and they accepted," he said. "And they accepted, they accepted."

He told me he had slept with at least eight women during retreats but that his only transgression was cheating on his wife. "I made my mistakes," he told me. "And I paid a price, I paid a steep price, and now I'm tired of suffering, of crying."

Victor said he sank into a deep depression after the November 2021 retreat and began seeing a therapist and undergoing hypnosis sessions to tame what he called his "powerful sexual energy."

He told me he had proof that Michelle was a liar and offered to send me an audio recording and transcript of conversations they had after Kailey posted her Facebook video.

In a November 20, 2021, text message, he begged Michelle to tell the other women he had not raped her. Michelle responded, "I already said what I had to say," and told him, "Don't write to me anymore please."

Victor replied, "Don't forget that karma is real and it will get you."

In the recorded phone call, Victor, sounding menacing, tells Michelle she needs to say their sex was consensual. I was stunned he deemed the exchange exculpatory and wanted to share it with me. In it, Michelle repeatedly asserts she sought to fend off his advances. "I told you from the beginning that I didn't want to do anything beyond being friends," she said.

Speaking about the sex act, she added in the call, "I told you no, I didn't want things to progress in that direction."

In the call, Victor tells Michelle that he was not himself those days. "I was sick, I was sick," he said. "Something possessed me." But, seconds later, seemingly contradicting himself, he argues that they both enjoyed the sex. "We both wanted it," he said. "We did it, we did it and we enjoyed—right?"

In a flat voice, she replied, "I sincerely didn't enjoy it. That's why I wanted it to stop."

As the retreat participants settled into their routines back home, Kailey and Tabatha felt strongly that Victor needed to be held accountable. They contacted the American embassy in Lima. Officials there informed them of a prominent warning in the State Department's travel advisory for Peru: "U.S. travelers participating in Ayahuasca and Kambo ceremonies should be aware that numerous persons, including U.S. citizens, have reported that while under the influence of these substances, they have witnessed or been victims of sexual assault, rape, theft, serious health problems and injuries, and even death." Kailey said officials at the embassy told them that in order to press charges, the women would have to hire a local attorney, then suggested a name. Kailey explored that possibility, but the lawyer demanded a $10,000 retainer and warned that the cost of taking Victor to court would be significant. "None of us have enough money to really contribute much toward the retainer," Kailey said.

Kailey asked the administrator of the Facebook group Kambo Kulture, which has more than eleven thousand members, for permission to publish an account of Victor's abuse. The administrator, she said, turned her down, afraid the allegations would have legal ramifications.

While Kailey and some of the other women debated how best to warn people about Victor, Michelle said her inclination was to put the whole ordeal behind her. Early on, she questioned whether the term *rape* was a fitting description of what happened. For months, she resisted using the term.

"It was really hard for me to accept that this was a part of my story," she said. "I didn't want to be seen as weak, and I didn't want to feel weak, most importantly."

Then she said something that took my breath away. On some level, she feels compassion toward Victor, whom she came to see as both a predator and a man with a genuine healing vocation.

"I know how heavy the word *rape* is and how it can ruin someone's life," she said. "I knew that in his heart of hearts he wanted to heal people, and I didn't want to take that away from him."

But nearly a year after the encounter, Michelle said she has come to feel entitled to use the term she long fought. "I feel like I can definitely say that it was an abuse of power, a lack of responsibility, accountability, and definitely rape," she said. "My energy felt very raped. My body felt raped."

Victor told me he feels like a broken man. He said he has no plans to resume running retreats and is focused on trying to salvage his relationship with Natasha.

"Did I err?" he said. "I did. And karma found me."

That glum mood did not last long. Within a few months, Victor and Natasha were again holding retreats in Peru and posting photos and videos of their latest guests on social media. One video shared on Facebook less than a year after my conversation with Victor shows him standing in the jungle holding a bright green frog with two young women standing next to him.

"Come to the Amazon to meet this frog," a smiling Victor says, looking at the camera. "He is a master. He is the medicine."

8 "BOOT CAMP HEALING"

The Ayahuasca Queer Retreat in Peru

THE FIRST TO BRING UP suicidal ideation was Fia Duda, who at twenty-four was the youngest among the twenty participants at the Temple of the Way of Light's inaugural retreat for queer people. It was our second day at the Temple, one of the oldest and most established ayahuasca centers in Peru, and we were sitting in a circle inside the maloca, introducing ourselves. The first few speakers kept their remarks short and relatively circumspect. But Fia didn't hesitate to tell us she had booked the retreat hoping it would put an end to the desire to kill herself. The nagging urge, which she first remembers feeling as an eight-year-old, had grown into a daily torment that intensified in the days leading up to the retreat. "I am trying to figure out why suicide is so baked in me," Fia said, speaking in a quiet but assured voice. "It's only gotten worse."

I scanned the room anticipating Fia's candor might spark a panicky reaction. Hearing someone speak about suicidal ideation induced a feeling of vertigo. I wondered whether the retreat organizers would pull Fia aside once we adjourned and tell her it would be unwise to go through the six ayahuasca ceremonies that awaited us during the twelve-day retreat. Surely there were protocols and red lines for situations like these. Subjecting someone in Fia's state to a blitz of tripping felt like playing shamanic Russian roulette. But instead of alarm, Fia's disclosure was met with compassionate, knowing gazes. They foreshadowed the disclosures that would emerge over the next few days as suicidality became a dominant theme of the retreat.

Before ceding the floor, Fia ended on as reassuring a note as she could muster. "I'm still here," she said, managing a slight smile. I didn't know it then, but sitting in silence were a handful of people who had come close to ending their lives. There was Holly Regan, a nonbinary journalist from the West Coast, who would later recount the day they woke up in the hospital room realizing the handful of pills they swallowed hadn't been enough to put an end to their misery. There was Ed, a redheaded nurse from England who just weeks earlier had hung a noose from his bathroom door, penned a farewell note, and then drank so heavily he passed out before going through with his plan. And, of course, there was me.

When I arrived in Peru for the retreat, it had been years since I had experienced suicidal ideation. But I walked into this experience with significant trepidation, having some major changes in the preceding months. For starters, I had left Brazil and moved to frosty Minnesota during the cruelest month of winter, to move in with Steve, the veterinarian. Stepping away from a regular job and routine for the first time in my adult life to focus on writing a book had begun to feel more disconcerting than liberating. And I sensed that the common thread that united the participants who signed up for this retreat would force me to wrestle with some demons I had kept on the back burner.

〰〰 The Temple opened in 2007 in a patch of thick jungle near Iquitos, the largest city in the world accessible only by riverboat and planes. There's a noisy casino with incandescent lights on virtually every block, and the roads are dominated by a mob of beeping, anarchic tuk-tuks, three-wheeled open vehicles, often packed to the brim.

The sweltering town has long been the gateway for people traveling to ayahuasca retreat centers like the Temple, which has become a shamanic proving ground where scores of facilitators—including Spring Washam—trained before going off to create competing franchises. The growing marketplace has done little to dampen the center's appeal. Retreats at the Temple, which offers comfortable, but decidedly austere, accommodations and plain food, often sell out more than six months in advance. Newer ayahuasca centers have sought to stand out by serving other psychoactive drugs in addition to ayahuasca, promising overnight transcendence, offering five-star lodging, and serving gourmet cuisine. But the Temple has remained understated in its marketing, presenting its program as more of a crucible than an adventure. It calls its protocol "boot camp healing," a marathon of sorts performed under the care of a team of taciturn Indigenous Shipibo healers trained in an ancestral form of energy cleansing.

The process has three stages. During an introductory ayahuasca ceremony, the Shipibo *curanderos* study each guest, whom they refer to as *pasajeros*, or passengers, to diagnose the nature and source of energetic blockages that are causing physical ailments, emotional distress, or both. During the subsequent ceremonies, the Shipibo maestros say they channel spirits from the plant world to intone piercing a cappella *icaros*. The songs are the main curative element within a ritual that also includes blowing tobacco smoke and spraying droplets of a sweet cologne known as *agua florida* on *pasajeros*. The aim is to dislodge *malos aires*, the negative energies that get trapped inside the body.

To draw them out, Shipibo healers often elicit violent purging during the ceremonies. Other tactics include daily steam baths scented with plants, bitter juices that are said to cleanse vital organs, and massages that tend to be more painful than soothing. The Shipibo spend the last few days of each retreat building a protective shield, known as an Arkana, for each *pasajero*. They describe it as an invisible screen meant to keep people from drawing negative energies and falling back into harmful patterns.

The morning before our first ceremony, we were introduced to the two maestros and two maestras who would oversee our care. Toni Lopez, the most outgoing among them, said that for the process to work, we needed to heed a couple of crucial instructions. During ceremonies, each *pasajero* would get a personalized *ícaro* from each of the maestros, who move around the round ceremony room counter-clockwise during the night, focusing on one person at a time. When a *pasajero* is being sung to, Toni said, he or she must sit upright, face the maestro, and do their utmost to rid the mind of thoughts. "You need to concentrate," he said. "You need to be in sync with us, with the plants, with the medicine." Toni said it would be tempting to get stuck in thinking loops, but doing so would only make their work harder. "The medicine will reveal many things," he went on. "But you need to stay focused." The second core instruction was just as important, he said. The process requires faith. "We don't want you to be doubting," he told us. "Just surrender."

As the meeting was wrapping up, Jeff, a Canadian participant, asked a question that had been on my mind: How do queer people fit within Shipibo culture? Toni dodged the question at first, saying only that they were "very happy" to be with us. I followed up, asking if there are same-sex couples in Shipibo communities and whether gay people were accepted. The maestros shared uncomfortable glances, and Toni stared at the floor for a few seconds before answering. "Before, there was a lot of discrimination," he finally conceded. Same-sex couples don't exist in Shipibo communities, he added, but stigma about people like us has receded. "Before, it was looked down on," he said. "But it can't be prohibited. Nature has a way of showing us how to evolve."

∿∿∿ The Temple was founded by Matthew Watherston, a British entrepreneur who stumbled into ayahuasca in early 2007 when he was navigating a midlife crisis. He signed up for ceremonies in Peru, hoping they would ease his crippling anxiety. But the experience did much more than that. Matthew said he walked away convinced that he was destined to establish a "healing facility" in the heart of the Amazon to treat people like him, beset with what he calls "twenty-first-century malaise, a sort of psycho-emotional black plague." Matthew was stepping into a complex world he knew little about. His partner in the venture, the Peruvian healer who introduced him to ayahuasca, stole much of the money Matthew wired to build the center, he said. Once it was up and running, he added, that healer and the other shamans he recruited sexually harassed the first female guests at the Temple. Just a few months after breaking ground, Matthew shut down the Temple, feeling it had become a sinister place under the spell of black magic. "It felt somewhat like *The Blair Witch Project*," he said. "This purpose, this calling, seemed to have crumbled." But soon after he returned home feeling defeated, a friend encouraged Matthew to meet a team of six elderly female Shipibo healers. Matthew hired the women as his new partners and set out to turn the Temple into the gold standard of ayahuasca retreats—an incubator of Shipibo healing traditions. In preserving this knowledge, Matthew saw an opportunity to make amends for the brutal legacy of colonialism in the Amazon basin. "Our forefathers extracted everything they could get their hands on—gold, rubber, minerals, oil," he said. "The last thing left is the wisdom of the medicines of the Amazon."

Over the past fifteen years, Matthew has worked with scores of Shipibo healers, participated in hundreds of ayahuasca ceremonies, and done several plant diets, periods of seclusion during which dieters consume little beyond a sacred plant they are trying to learn from. Yet the nature of the Shipibo healing process remains largely mysterious to him. "It's incomprehensible; it exists beyond the mind," Matthew said. "Our minds cannot figure out and understand healing from a shamanic perspective, and they're not supposed to." The nature of our thinking minds is at the root of our suffering. "We're never going to resolve issues and problems from the same level of thinking that created them in the first place," Matthew said. "It can only be understood through experience." I asked how he would describe his own. "What I slowly began to understand is that what this system is doing is peeling back layer upon layer of illusions that I had identified with as constituting who I am," he said. "Now, where was that illusion derived from? Essentially, trauma." Over years, Matthew said, it's possible to peel off those layers of trauma, one by one, which leaves us with a sense of self that is lighter, less burdened by the past.

〜〜 From our first day at the Temple, it was clear we were undergoing a collective unburdening. There was something profoundly liberating about being in a community of queer people. It loosened up our body language, which so many of us have been conditioned to modulate to heteronormative standards in the pursuit of safety and acceptance. We spoke with striking candor about sex, relationships, and loneliness. We discussed our love-hate relationships with hookup apps, at once so convenient and dehumanizing. We shared views on our relationship with pornography. Many of us were physically affectionate, getting lost in long, sometimes tearful embraces. It felt comfortable to hold hands, rest your head on someone's lap— gestures that felt especially nourishing in a rare queer environment in which sex was explicitly off the table.

But to me, the most transgressive feature of this queer psychedelic bubble we found ourselves in was how easily frank conversations about suicidality emerged, both in group and one-on-one conversations. We all knew, on some level, that suicidal ideation is chillingly common among queer people. A 2022 mental health survey by the Trevor Project, which provides crisis intervention to young queer people, found that 45 percent of LGBTQ youth between the ages of thirteen and twenty-four had seriously considered killing themselves. Among transgender and nonbinary youth, the crisis is more severe: one in five have attempted to end their lives, according to the survey. At the Temple, it dawned on me that I had never previously had a revealing conversation about suicidal ideation. I had intentionally steered clear of bringing up my own during therapy. And it never occurred to me to ask close friends whether it was a

demon they had wrestled with. There are good reasons for this. Yana
Calou, one of the participants of the retreat, has spent much of their
career thinking about them. Yana, who is nonbinary, is the director
of advocacy at Trans Lifeline, a peer support and crisis hotline run
by and for transgender people. They told me suicidal people are often reluctant to seek help because intervention responses can have
severe and destabilizing consequences. Due diligence responses by
a therapist, an employer, or a hotline operator can set in motion a
police response, an involuntary hospitalization. Resisting can lead a
despondent person to jail. Those who comply can face huge medical
bills, getting fired, and losing custody of children. People at each step
of the intervention system may mean well, Yana said, but their efforts
seldom add up to a holistic response that addresses the root causes
of a person's despair. "The research on queer and trans people has
been really clear about what's making us have suicide attempt and
ideation rates that are through the roof," Yana said. "There's a huge
lack of care, support, community, love, and belonging that each of
us experience."

The application form for a Temple retreat inquires whether an ap-
plicant has attempted suicide in the past and whether they are actively experiencing ideation. I asked Públio Valle, a veteran facilitator
at the Temple who led our retreat, how the team there has come
to think about suicidality among participants. Públio, a tall, lanky
Brazilian who has a gentle, monk-like demeanor, told me that acute
suicidality can be disqualifying if facilitators determine that a retreat
is likely to do more harm than good. But over the years, Públio said,
he has found value in meeting mentions of suicidality with warmth
and empathy rather than alarm. "When I hear of someone being
suicidal, the first thing that comes to mind is: there's so much pain
there that it's unbearable and this person is trying to find a way out
of this pain," he said. "If we give space and support for that person
to get in touch with the discomfort, with the layers of pain that are
inside, there is a relief, and that urgent need to escape, that discomfort, subsides."

Públio's colleague Juliana Bizare told me that she doesn't think we'll ever understand, on a rational level, how ayahuasca brings about profound changes. But one thing she has come to see clearly is that it often upends a person's understanding of the healing process and their role within it. In the Western medical system, she said, patients are conditioned to be passive and deferential to medical professionals. Interventions often address symptoms while overlooking causes of disease and distress. The Shipibo system demands much more from patients, who often come to see clearly patterns of behavior and sources of pain that can be addressed through hard and sustained work. "When I work with people, I have a deep trust in their capacity for healing," she said. "Otherwise, I would not do this work, because we see so much pain and suffering."

〰〰 Early in my newspaper career, I learned that we typically steer clear of covering suicides, based on the theory that drawing attention to them can encourage people to kill themselves. We're told to use nonstigmatizing language when we write about them. An obituary will note that someone *died by suicide*, a phrasing that always struck me as odd, steering clear of the word *committed*, a loaded and accusatory verb. The takeaway is that public discussions of suicide ought to be euphemistic and infrequent. Yet I had stumbled into the rare setting in which people were more than willing to speak about this darkest of impulses. The long conversations that began at the retreat and continued in the months that followed convinced me that creating more space for these discussions can help those who live with suicidal ideation feel less alone and misunderstood.

Holly, the nonbinary journalist, told me their thoughts of suicide began after their parents separated when they were eight. Self-harm impulses intensified over the years as Holly, who was raised by a devout evangelical mother, began feeling sexual urges that felt transgressive.

"I already thought I was going to hell for being attracted to women," they told me. "Well, I'm definitely going to hell if I kill myself."

For years, Holly tempted death with reckless behavior. "I drove drunk everywhere and had so many accidents; I almost died so many times," Holly said. That inclination toward self-harm took a dangerous form on a sunny Fourth of July gathering at a friend's backyard in Austin. After getting into a loud fight with a boyfriend, Holly retreated to a shady spot under a tree and gulped down a fistful of ibuprofen. Fading in and out of consciousness, Holly remembers seeing a chirping bird land on a tree branch right above their head. *Oh shit,* Holly recalls thinking. *I've actually done it this time.* Then came a panicky thought. *I don't want to never see birds again. I have to see trees again. I want to live!*

Holly managed to get up, walked unsteadily toward their partner, and let him know what they had done. The partner had found the body of his brother, who died by suicide years earlier, Holly said. Holly said the sequence of events that came next are a blur, but they involve an ambulance ride and waking up in a small hospital room realizing their wrists were strapped down. When a nurse popped into the room, Holly stammered that they wanted to go home. "Yeah, well, you tried to kill yourself," Holly recalled the nurse saying. "So we can't do that." Over the next twelve hours or so, Holly pleaded to be allowed to leave, but each protestation triggered a fresh injection of a sedative into an IV line in their arm.

Days after leaving the Temple, Holly told me they experienced a moment of eureka involving the strained relationship with their father. Exactly how it happened remains mysterious, said Holly, who told me they had been able to forgive him and make peace with painful aspects of their childhood. With the easing of such a long-standing source of torment, Holly found themself incandescently happy to be alive. "I'm going to be super cliché," Holly said in a video they broadcast live on social media the day before leaving Peru. "I've just had a spiritual awakening."

〰 I did a double take when Ed revealed during one of our group meetings that he had come close to hanging himself earlier in the year. He was hilarious and warm in equal measure, and I had been drawn to him from the first day. This was his third time at the Temple, he said; he'd felt the urge to return after a recent breakup with a longtime partner. There was nothing in Ed's demeanor that conveyed distress. The ease with which he made people laugh made it easy to assume he was a fundamentally happy person. Which was why eyes widened and jaws dropped when Ed revealed this.

"Just a few weeks ago, I got a bit drunk, drank a box of wine, and woke up the next day to find I had written a suicide note," he told us in a quivering voice. "I don't remember writing it."

Ed remembered that he had intended to hang himself in his bathroom before blacking out from drinking. The note he penned was brief and not abrupt: "I'm so sorry but this hasn't worked," he wrote. "I can't make life work for whatever reason."

Speaking barely above a whisper, Ed shared painful memories about his father. He had so often been cruel, Ed said, prone to subjecting his family to depraved pranks. One day, he put a dead pig in the passenger's side of the car to scare Ed's mother. Once, as a form of punishment, he locked Ed and his brother outside the home during a freezing winter night so long their skin turned blue. During outbursts of anger, he could chase Ed and his brother through the house, brandishing a whip, as the boys ran to the only bathroom in the house with a lock. "All these memories showed up, of not being protected," Ed said.

As an adult, he said, he felt he carried a form of "darkness" that felt impossible to shake. Thoughts of suicide had been a constant since he was a teenager, he later told me. "I didn't think I would kill myself, because of what it would do to my mom," he said. "But I figured I would just go through life as a ghost, as the walking dead, and drink myself to death."

Ed said that something profound had shifted within him during the last two ceremonies. Much of it could not be put into words. But one of the main insights was about intergenerational trauma. "I came to the understanding that the people who traumatized me were traumatized themselves," he said. "It was wrong that it happened, but part of me could not blame them." Ed told me he had first gone to the Temple in 2014 because he had been an "unhappy person" for as long as he could remember. Beyond the abuse at home, he was bullied and assaulted at school. And he struggled to connect intimately and sexually with partners. He walked away from the initial retreat with an unfamiliar feeling. "Life seemed brighter," he explained. "And it was only by having that taste of brightness that I realized how dark things had gotten."

Over the years, Ed said, he has come to see the people who hurt him with compassion. And he has come to see forgiveness as the most healing act—albeit one that often unfolds slowly and haltingly. "I used to think forgiveness was like an on-and-off switch, and I felt ashamed if I could not forgive someone," he said. "But forgiveness is something you do moment by moment, day by day; it can be two steps forward, three steps back."

He has thought long and hard about his parents' generation, he told me, baby boomers in the United Kingdom who had to "metabolize the trauma of the war" during an era in which mental illness was seldom discussed, let alone treated. "Now we're having to process our own trauma," he said. "And to some degree, we're having to metabolize the trauma of the generation before at the same time."

Ed said he had been uneasy about coming on a queer retreat, fearing it would make him confront raw feelings that didn't come to the surface during previous ones. "The thing that struck me was the shame, the collective shame," he said. "These days with all the progress and all the Netflix shows, it's easy to think the war has been won." But there was a striking degree of overlap in the personal narratives that unspooled over our twelve days at the Temple, Ed said. And there was something liberating and enthralling about bonding with other gay men in an environment where no one was pursuing sex. "I found real joy luxuriating in that true connection," he said. "It wasn't about who's getting off with who but about resting your head on somebody's shoulder, crying with someone, opening up with others who felt ashamed of their bodies."

During his time at the Temple, Ed said, he came to think differently about his suicidal ideation. "In one ceremony, I had an image of the pain and suffering and negativity within me, and it was like a dying animal and it was screaming, and part of me didn't want to let it go." But he did—somehow. "I feel like a part of me died in the jungle," he said. "It was a part of me that was ready to go."

〰 Midway through the retreat, I sat next to Fia during lunch one day. There was something confounding about her appearance, at once youthful and weathered. She has piercing blue eyes and a movie star smile. Her blond hair is in dreads, and much of her body, including her forehead, is covered in tattoos. When Fia mentioned in passing that her father had killed himself just a few years earlier, I became curious about her upbringing. Her suicidal ideation began when she was eight, Fia told me. The catalyst was an explosive fight between her parents that led to Fia's mother getting arrested. The years that followed were a blur of depression as she bounced between a school where she was the target of malicious gossip and a dysfunctional home. Desperately yearning to die, Fia figured the only realistic means at her disposal was to starve herself. "I never actually attempted, other than starving myself," she said. "That became my drawn-out, long-term goal."

In her late teens, Fia moved in with her father, who lived in Tampa and had struggled with addiction for most of his life. She became something of a caretaker for her dad, who drank heavily and was hooked on opioids. He cycled in and out of rehab, never managing to stay clean for long. At home, he constantly brought up how badly he wanted to die. "Every single day, he would say, 'I'm going to kill myself,'" Fia recalled. "It was almost like the boy who cried wolf because you hear it so many times."

Early on the morning of December 12, 2015, Fia and her father got into a fight after she fell asleep on the living room couch. Her father had been acting particularly deranged that week, she said. When he threatened to kill himself—again—Fia said something that would haunt her for years. Just above a whisper, she said, "Well, why don't you do it?"

That afternoon, as she was getting ready to leave school and head to her job waiting tables at an Asian restaurant, a friend pulled Fia aside to share some shocking news. Cops were outside her house. Neighbors had heard a gunshot inside. Her father was presumed dead.

The facts didn't register. "I didn't believe it," she told me, so she headed to work, unwilling to absorb the news. But soon, a police officer called her cell phone and urged her to come home immediately to unlock the door. Sure enough, inside they found her dad in a pool of blood, having died from a self-inflicted gunshot wound.

As she grieved his loss, Fia retreated from the world. She was tormented by the thought that she may have pushed her father over the edge with those muffled words. "For a long time, I thought maybe he had heard me, and that was, like, just the push he needed to go through with it."

Fia said that her father's death effectively took suicide off the table as an option for her because she realized the devastation such a death leaves in its wake. But the thoughts only intensified.

I asked Fia how her thoughts about her father's passing had shifted over the years. Her answer surprised me. "I saw my dad suffering my whole life, so I now see his choice of taking his life as a gift he was giving himself," she said. It may seem odd, Fia added, but she now thinks it was the best outcome for both of them. "If he was still here today, it sounds awful to say, but he would be a burden for me," she said. It was a searingly honest answer, the kind people seldom speak out loud.

Something unexpected happened in the weeks after Fia left Peru. Her suicidal ideation receded almost entirely for the first time in her adult life, she said. She found herself forming close bonds with people and leaning into long-term goals. "When you're suicidal, you drop everything that you ever thought you could or wanted to do," she said. "You really have to make an effort finding meaning in things and having a lust for life because you have been clouded for so long that you forgot there was something out there to live for."

〰〰 I did more listening than speaking during conversations about suicide in Peru. But during the next-to-last ceremony of the retreat, I had an intense experience that would change that. It began with a burst of vivid memories from the years I spent covering conflicts in Iraq, Afghanistan, and Libya. The scenes flashed before my eyes like vivid dreams, startling me with the level of detail that somehow endured in dark corners of my mind all these years. But this string of recollections, which followed a clear theme, was suddenly interrupted by a far older memory that had been shelved for decades. I saw myself in a small, windowless room with a stale smell, sitting on the edge of a bed, one of three naked bodies. Lying on the bed is a tired-looking sex worker with stretch marks on her belly and small, sagging breasts. I watch as a high school classmate, JP, bites into the edge of a condom wrapper, rolls the rubber back on his penis. Sharing a sex worker with him was my idea. It took several weeks of meticulous planning to get him to agree, to figure out the brothel marketplace in Bogotá, and to settle on a price and a date. Having gotten my way on something I desperately yearned for, I'm suddenly in agony. The unspoken rules are crystal clear. We take turns having sex with her, but steer clear of even incidental skin-on-skin contact between us. The rules chafe because all I want to do is disregard this woman, who seems amused by our glaring inexperience, and press his warm body against mine. But I suppress this urge and wallow in the deep shame I'd carry within for years.

Without warning, I zoom out of that dank room with its lumpy mattress and yellowed sheets, and find myself on the hilly streets of San Francisco. It is morning, and fog lingers over the bay. I am walking alone toward the Golden Gate Bridge, wearing white sneakers that lurch forward in long, determined strides. I am a man on a mission. It suddenly occurs to me that, unlike the previous ones, this is not a memory in my inventory. Those shoes were never mine. I've visited San Francisco briefly a couple of times, but experienced nothing meaningful or traumatic there. So I try to zoom out, like someone who has accidentally popped into the wrong meeting room. This is clearly a mistake. But my efforts to direct my focus to a familiar memory, to exit this dreamlike state, are for naught. As I give in to this delusion, a feeling of vertigo sets in. The realization takes hold slowly, but I start to sense where this is going, and it feels irrevocable. I have questions, and I ask them breathlessly, as though there is a sentient being directing this strange scene, as though there is an escape hatch to be found. It is conveyed that this is not me but a past life, a concept that up to this point I had not believed in, ruled out, or given much thought to. I ask for a name but don't get it. I ask if the man is going to jump. *Just watch*, I'm told. And so I do, with restless resignation. I keep putting one foot in front of the other. It is vivid and panic-inducing like a nightmare, but different, because I am awake and aware of being so. As I make it to the bridge, I realize Anita, the tiny, elderly maestra, has plopped down next to me. I question my ability to sit up and face her, but with considerable effort, I manage to pull my head off the mat. The first notes of her song are soft but penetrating, discordant but assured. As her *icaro* quickens, the feet come to a halt. I am roughly at the midsection of the bridge. I see a pair of hands clasp onto the railings. And suddenly the fear of jumping, of surrendering to the lethal force of gravity for a few agonizing seconds, subsides. I very much want to jump. One leg swings over the railing. Then the other. A quick scan to the right and the left confirms there will be no witnesses, no one to intervene, no hero to save the day. I loosen the muscles in my fingers and tumble toward the water, a mass of despair about to meet its end. My body jolts at the point of impact, but there is no pain. Anita has stopped singing and is shifting unsteadily to the next mat. And so I let my head fall back into the mat and lie there in astonished wonder.

When the ceremony finally came to an end, I stumbled back to my room under the glow of a bright moon. My first instinct was to discard this chilling scene as one of meaningless musings and delusions that ayahuasca inflicts on a weary mind. But the memory remained vivid and tantalizing when I awoke from a few hours of sleep. I could still feel the vertigo that came as the hand ungripped the railing, the silent seconds of free fall, at once terrifying and liberating. The jolt at the end—an irreversible crossing into a domain unknown.

〰️ For the next couple of days, I wrestled with how to interpret the suicide vision. I feared I was breathing life into an unhealthy death wish that my mind kept replaying on a loop. It was tempting to think that I had unlocked a layer of knowledge about the roots of my suffering. How liberating it would be to come to believe that much of the pain and dread that weighs us down predates this bodily existence. Could a past life that ended suddenly on that bridge be an important thread of the tapestry of symptoms I had come to call depression? And if so, was there a way to untether my suffering from the man who flung his body off the bridge? One of the marvels of ayahuasca retreats is you can raise questions as bizarre as these without fear of being laughed at or institutionalized.

On a sunny afternoon, I sat down with Toni, who was the chattiest among the *curanderos*, and asked him if he believed in past lives. I suddenly found myself less ambivalent on the matter, and I desperately wanted validation that what I had experienced had meaning and purpose. But Toni's response was disappointing.

"After death, a large bird comes and collects a person's spirit," he said. "They go to a place below the earth and remain there, tranquil." The dead remain accessible to people who develop spiritual powers, but there's no path for them to come back in human form.

Then I asked Toni what he made of the people in our group and whether there was anything distinct about us. He took a deep breath. "I'm going to tell you the truth," he finally said. The scale of self-loathing and pain the *curanderos* picked up from our group was striking, he said as the two female *curanderas* sitting beside him nodded. "These are people with good hearts, but many have been rejected by their families, by society," he went on. "Some aren't loved by their parents, and that leaves a very profound type of pain."

I asked Toni if there is an antidote to that type of pain. The answer, he said, was at once simple and extraordinarily complex. "We must learn to think less." I asked him to elaborate. Toni said there are three stages in life: the past, the present moment, and the future. Suffering stems from a tendency to ruminate incessantly about the past, far beyond what is useful to heed its lessons, and to fret about the future, getting caught up in loops of indecision. "We must learn to live in the present moment," he said. "The past is in the past." Regarding the future, Toni said, it's necessary to be at once optimistic and decisive, "without fear or doubt."

〰〰 A few months after leaving Peru, I went to the wedding of a high school classmate from Colombia and saw the friend with whom I had once shared a sex worker. JP had a receding hairline but the same playful, jokester demeanor that had made him attractive to me when we were teenagers. He now works producing reality cooking shows in Los Angeles, where he is married to a woman and raising two kids. During the rehearsal dinner, he pulled me aside after he was a few drinks in and said it troubled him deeply that we had drifted apart over the years, that I had become something of a recluse. "I *love* you, Ernie," he said, using a nickname that thankfully didn't stick after high school. He asked why I had effectively cut off all my high school friends. I told him I had a strange story to share and recounted the memory of our sexual escapade, explaining it had surfaced in vivid detail during an ayahuasca ceremony. "Raquel!" he exclaimed, surprising me by remembering the woman's name. I told him I felt that I had been manipulative in arranging the encounter and feared that after I came out of the closet he may have come to see my behavior as predatory. JP looked stunned. "We were kids," he said. "We did crazy things." He said he didn't think I had acted maliciously, then or now, and that he was sorry we hadn't had a chance to clear the air all these years. He pulled me into an embrace and said it was not too late to salvage our friendship.

I had been acquitted of a transgression that had existed only in my mind. I let my body sink into his for a few seconds as people danced around us. "I love you too," I said.

9   CHASING MIRACLES IN COSTA RICA

THE FIRST TWO THINGS THAT caught my eye as the taxi was allowed inside the gates of Rythmia Life Advancement Center were the helipad just outside the lobby and the golf carts. I had barely stepped out of the car when a handful of young men dressed in immaculate white uniforms swarmed around me and guided me through the check-in process with clockwork precision. One handed me a fragrant, moist white towel. Another handed me a white Rythmia tote bag that contained a Rythmia water bottle, a Rythmia shot glass, and a workbook titled *THE RYTHMIA WAY*, which outlined the busy schedule for the week ahead.

I was then handed a stack of documents, including a RELEASE OF LIABILITY form on which my last name was misspelled. Signers were asked to acknowledge that "while engaging in the activities offered by Rythmia there is the heightened possibility of physical harm," but by signing the document, they are "forever releasing Rythmia its heirs and assigns from any reasons regarding my general health and well-being." Had they had a lawyer draft this? I wondered. Hell, had a literate human proofread it? The form continued: anyone who decided to sue Rythmia despite the aforementioned needed to agree that all matters would be "resolved under Costa Rican law and all disputes will be heard and argued in Guanacaste, Costa Rica." I provided an emergency contact name and number at the end of the form and signed my name with more than a bit of trepidation.

I was quickly guided to an adjacent office, where a young man took my photo and gave me a white wristband with an electronic chip. Every building at Rythmia is outfitted with a scanning device. Guests are asked to swipe their wristbands every time they enter and leave a class, workshop, and ceremony, in order to keep track of attendance at "mandatory" and "optional" sessions in the schedule that starts with yoga at 7:00 a.m. and ends with ayahuasca ceremonies that sometimes last until dawn. In a letter at the beginning of the workbook, Rythmia founder Gerard Powell urges guests not to skip the first mandatory session held on Monday mornings, titled: "About Your Miracle." The session, sometimes led by Gerry himself, is a dramatic rendition of how tripping on an African plant called iboga a few years ago set in motion Gerry's miraculous transformation. In the blink of an eye, he went from being a miserable, suicidal, wife-beating, loathsome multimillionaire addicted to drugs, alcohol, and sex to a man who would address incoming guests at his luxury "plant medicine" resort as "Dear Friend in Spirit." Gerry's letter continued: "My sole purpose in this life is to make sure that each participant at Rythmia receives a life changing miracle during their stay." But in order to "ensure the highest likelihood of this occurrence in your life, you need to attend my two-hour discussion titled: 'About Your Miracle & Introduction to Plant Medicine.'"

The final steps at check-in were to book a massage and two Dead Sea Cleanses, which is the Rythmia name for colonics. As I was handed the key to a room I would share with a mystery roommate, I noticed an LED banner sign that read: "Miracle rate: 97.20. Today's forecast YOURS IS HAPPENING :)" I let out an incredulous chortle as I walked through the resort's beautifully landscaped gardens, which are adorned with enormous Buddha statues.

As I made my way to the orientation class, the first mandatory session of the week, I took in the chic beach-vacation fashion statements; there were panama hats, linen pants, and, among women, generously applied makeup and more than a few fake eyelashes.

This was the first retreat I was attending first and foremost as a journalist. My goal was to document ayahuasca rituals catering to the 1 percent. It's a share of the market that has found a sweet spot in Costa Rica, which has just the right blend of exotic, safe, and accessible to entice the kind of traveler who might find the Amazon too far, too foreign, too rustic, and too mystical.

Since its founding in 2016, Rythmia has become among the most popular and controversial centers in the medicinal psychedelic field. Promoting itself as a "medically-licensed plant medicine center," it caters to as many as ninety guests at once, while competitors try to keep groups small and intimate. Its marketing strategy relies heavily on C-list celebrities, bro-ey podcasters, and #blessed Instagram influencers. While most ayahuasca retreat organizers cater to people in need of healing, Rythmia guarantees a miracle to every guest who is obsequious and credulous. It offers up Gerry's asshole-to-healer journey as a template of what's attainable in the healing marketplace for those who can plunk down $6,000 on a weeklong retreat. I would soon learn that virtually every Rythmia employee has a Gerry-like Hero's Journey, and a penchant to share a ton about what a train wreck their lives were before they collided with Gerry's—in miraculous synchronicity.

"How many of you already had synchronicities before coming here?" Bernie Gonzalez, the Rythmia employee who ran our orientation class, asked the tightly packed room, flashing a knowing smile. I caught several blank stares and a few enthusiastic nods. "It's all cosmic magic," Bernie said. "You were supposed to be here."

Then Bernie launched into her personal story, the first of what would become a familiar yarn delivered with dramatic flair, well-rehearsed punch lines, and an amount of cursing that felt transgressive in a pseudo-spiritual enclave. Bernie told us she used to be a highly effective cog in the capitalist matrix, working a senior finance job at Nissan. It made her sick, as the corporate world is prone to do, and a physical ailment led to an emotional one. Talk therapy was useless, as were antidepressants and every conventional tool she tried until the day the internet algorithms delivered her a video of Gerry. Within weeks, she was on a flight to Liberia, Costa Rica. "I couldn't get here fast enough," she said. Bernie likened her week at Rythmia to being "beaten with a truth stick" and said she discovered how much of her suffering was inherited. "Your issues are in your tissues!" she exclaimed. Last year, her life's purpose became clear when Gerry offered her a job at Rythmia. Healing—herself and others—became a full-time labor of love, she said.

In order to have the kind of awakening she embodied, Bernie told us, it was imperative to "surrender to the medicine, because when you do, she will heal your heart." She warned that some of the things we would hear and feel and experience in the days ahead would be hard, confounding, and even maybe triggering. "You're going to be hearing about past lives and aliens," she said. "The impossible becomes possible." But it was vital to trust the system. "Those of you who were sleepwalking, like I was, become conscious, awake."

〜〜 The next morning, the first full day of the retreat, we gathered back in the same room and were jolted awake by John Jacob Mubarak, the Rythmia staffer who had been tasked with telling us Gerry's miracle story. Before launching into the yarn, JJ got the crowd loose and laughing with a handful of jokes. Teasingly inquiring about past drug use, he called cocaine users "my people," drawing hysterical laughter. Then he made the first of several cult jokes we would hear throughout the week, a trope that seemed designed to convey that members of an actual cult would never use the c-word, even in jest. "I haven't spoken to my family in six years, and all I do is pray to a picture of Gerry," JJ said as we all giggled.

The session, "About Your Miracle," is a centerpiece of the Rythmia week, presenting Gerry's story as a model of how we should aspire to heal in the days ahead, following a tightly prescriptive playbook. When Rythmia launched, Gerry, an engaging public speaker, normally delivered the talk. But now he largely relegates the task to deputies like JJ, who enthrall audiences by simultaneously trashing and lionizing the boss. I was familiar with Gerry's story, having read his memoir, *Sh*t the Moon Said: A Story of Sex, Drugs, and Ayahuasca*. JJ warned us again that much of what we were about to hear, during his talk and later in the week, would seem bonkers, triggering, and even appalling. But that was part of the process, he assured us. "Comfort is the goal, but not necessarily the means," he said. But he argued that it would be a waste of time and thousands of dollars to have made it all the way to Rythmia with a skeptic's mindset. "The difference between ninety-nine percent and one hundred percent is life-changing," he said. "So I'm going to ask you to be one hundred percent in! Are you all in?" The response was an emphatic roar of yeses. JJ said he knew it can be hard to trust, but he told us to reflect on words he attributed to the American abolitionist Harriet Tubman. "Harriet Tubman said she could have saved so many more people, but they didn't believe it was possible," JJ said. "They were scared, and for good reason."

But we had the chance to break free from the chains of depression and a sleepwalking existence, JJ assured us. "You have to believe with all your heart and all your soul that you can heal, that it's possible, and you will receive your miracle," he said. "You just have to trust and surrender and show up to the classes."

I found the Tubman quote captivating, and it made me question whether my resolute skepticism of the Rythmia way was self-defeating. I pulled out my phone to find the original quote. Instead, I found a short Associated Press article debunking the assertion, which had circulated widely in online memes. "False Quote on Freed Slaves Wrongly Attributed to Harriet Tubman," the headline read. It quoted abolition-era historians who said Tubman never said she could have freed more slaves if only they had believed it was possible. Skepticism intact, I sat back to take in JJ's eminently enjoyable rendition of the story of Gerry.

∿∿ Gerard Powell was born in Scranton, Pennsylvania, on September 21, 1963. After being expelled from one high school and dropping out of another, he began a series of ventures, including a telemarketing company, a real estate firm, and a plastic surgery company. He did well. But his management style was ruthless, his personal relationships a mess, and as his fortune grew, so did his distress. By the time he sold his last company for $89 million in 2004, Gerry writes, he had five homes, two planes, twenty-three cars, and a racehorse. "I had achieved the American dream—and then some— but I also knew something was very wrong," he wrote. "The more stuff I acquired, the more I suffered." He made those around him miserable, JJ said. "He became a real asshole, a womanizer, a wife-beater, an alcoholic, a drug addict, a cheat, a liar, a thief," JJ told us. "He had the kind of energy that people would move away from him at the CVS."

Gerry's substance abuse problems got worse after his father died in 2006, and he began injecting himself with Demerol, an opioid, daily. Finally, he decided to check into Passages, a luxurious rehab facility in Malibu, after a final four-day bender in a hotel room with an ex-girlfriend and "enough morphine to kill us both," he wrote.

After checking out of Passages, Gerry hired one of the center's psychologists, Jeff McNairy, to be his full-time shrink, and became reasonably functional for a few years, if never quite sober or happy. But another big unraveling came in 2014, when he got into a big fight with a girlfriend as they were preparing to board a flight to the Philippines. Gerry ripped up her ticket, dumped her, and checked into a couples' resort, alone. There, he made a woe-is-me Facebook post, which happened to be seen by a Passages alum, who happened to be in the Philippines and who happened to know just what Gerry needed to snap out of his downward spiral.

"Listen, Gerry, I had a friend who was just like you," the woman told Gerry. "He went to Costa Rica and did plant medicine, and when he came back, he was a completely different guy."

Gerry booked a spot on a retreat the woman recommended. Within days, he found himself in the garage of a beat-down house run by a shaman from Gabon named Moughenda, who administers ibogaine, a powerful psychedelic derived from an African plant. After taking ibogaine, Gerry says he left his body and traveled to the moon, where Moughenda said Gerry would find answers about the roots of his distress.

What followed, under the influence of the drug, was a conversation with the moon, the discovery that he had been sexually molested by his grandfather, a confrontation with the long-dead man, and finally, forgiveness. After that, Gerry said, he pulled out his heart, by then a black "pumice stone." The moon polished it up and returned it to him, perfect, "bright red and beating."

After slipping it back into his chest, Gerry made his way down from the moon and back into his body in Costa Rica—born again.

∿∿∿ During subsequent trips with Moughenda, the moon instructed Gerry to drop all his business pursuits—including his latest idea, a network of strip clubs in airports—and build a state-of-the-art healing center in Costa Rica. If iboga had been Gerry's salvation, I wondered, why on earth had Gerry ended up opening an ayahuasca retreat? JJ anticipated my question before I had a chance to ask it. "The moon told him, 'I want you to work with ayahuasca,'" JJ said, because it's a "gentler, more feminine energy."

The moral of Gerry's story, repeated throughout the week as gospel, is that there's a path to healing and redemption, even for the most sinful and broken among us. Furthermore, that path can be wildly entertaining and doesn't require a monastic existence.

To replicate Gerry's success, we needed to follow his playbook with diligent devotion. There are three steps. First step is to make a request of the moon—God, or ayahuasca, or whoever has some bandwidth for the pain of mortals up there in the cosmic realm—a fundamental question: *Show me who I have become.* According to Rythmia dogma, that inquiry inevitably leads to a highly unpleasant diagnosis and ultimately to a revelation. Guests discover they became miserable and sick as a result of a traumatic event in their childhood that made them disassociate, or part ways with their soul. Once there's a theory about when the soul and the body came undone, guests are instructed to move on to step two: ask for divine intervention to "merge me back with my soul—*at all costs.*" Once the soul merger is complete, the last and final step is to ask for a new heart, so you can be just like Gerry.

If this all sounded too good to be true, JJ said that skepticism was entirely normal and it often deepened as people put their bodies and minds through a marathon of tripping during four consecutive days without getting much sleep. "If you're doing this right, at some point you're going to go: *Get me the fuck out of here,*" he told us. "But that's actually a good thing. It means you're on the verge of a breakthrough—you're very, very close." The trick to overriding skepticism, he said, was to take full advantage of Rythmia's open-bar approach to serving ayahuasca—an anomaly in a field where dosing people carefully and judiciously is the norm. If we had the wherewithal to get up for another cup, JJ advised, we should. "Don't think, drink," he said, repeating it as a mantra. "The invitation is to push yourself a little more than you want to because no one ever mastered anything by being comfortable."

〰 I drank just one cup during the first ceremony, turning down the invitation to be uncomfortable. But most people heeded the call to chug down ayahuasca with abandon, and when the ceremony came to a close, a handful of them declared, in slurring and largely nonsensical sentences, that they had merged with their souls. The declarations were met with rapturous applause, which created a palpable sense of FOMO among the miracle-deprived in the group.

The next morning, having slept for less than two hours, I dragged myself to a yoga class at 7:00 a.m. It was taught by a comically chipper instructor who, like everyone else at Rythmia, delivered tried-and-tested, reasonably funny jokes as he led us through a gentle practice. His signature line, "¡No pasa nada!"—"Let it roll off!"—became a mantra people in the room were reciting with glee after every chaturanga. Despite being groggy from the night before, it dawned on me as I flickered in and out of sleep in savasana that this exuberant form of performative joy, which seemed to be a job requirement at Rythmia, was highly effective. Effervescent happiness can be a magnet for people who have spent long periods in the clutches of depression. And all around me, I saw fellow guests mirror the gleeful spirit on display, tuning in to a frequency in which logic is immaterial and doubt evaporates.

A case in point was the first workshop of the day, a session called "The Answer is You!"—taught by Kim Stanwood Terranova, a thin blond woman affiliated with the Agape International Spiritual Center in Beverly Hills. The church was founded by the Reverend Michael Beckwith, one of the most prominent evangelists of the law of attraction, which holds that you can think yourself into a life of abundance, health, and wild riches. Kim stopped often during her presentation to pray, asking "spirit" to help her answer questions people in the audience had asked. She spoke in a singsongy voice as she said things like "We're all swimming in an ocean of devotion together" and "There is so much light in your body temple." Having dabbled a bit in positive thinking, I found her theories of a life well lived, the power of positive thinking, and our relationship with fear harmless, even thought-provoking at times. But after she took a bow, she ceded the stage to a speaker that made my skepticism about Rythmia turn to horror.

It was a marketing presentation for one of Rythmia's add-ons, an intravenous injection of umbilical cord blood stem cells that are offered exclusively to guests during the final two days of the retreat. Before getting into the pseudoscience underpinning of NovaCell, as the product was called, the presenter, Alana Lambert, warmed up the crowd with a joke about nuns and anal sex before getting down to business.

The procedure on offer at Rythmia, she acknowledged, was not approved by the Food and Drug Administration and was not legal in the United States. But we ought to interpret that as a validation rather than a problem, she argued, because the American medical regulatory system was rigged by underhanded actors who profit from keeping people chronically ill. "The only people they make money off, Big Pharma, are sick people," she said. "If you're healthy, they can't make money off of you. If you're dead, they can't make money off of you. Big Pharma is a big business, and they want you sick."

Alana said that being injected with millions of stem cells collected from umbilical cords at a Costa Rican clinic "unlocks an almost limitless array of healing powers" by reducing inflammation and revitalizing organs. The fresh stem cells, she said, are drawn to parts of the body that are in distress. "Basically, you've got a stem cell here and it's kind of on its last legs, and then this brand-new stem cell comes in and is like: *Wake up!*" Alana explained. "And so your stem cells start acting like the new stem cells."

Alana said stem cell therapy had worked wonders for her parents, who had visited her earlier in the year, fearing their daughter "had joined a cult when I started working here." Her mother had long suffered from sciatica. Her father had REM disorder, a condition in which people physically act out their dreams, which can be dangerous. Both conditions vastly improved after getting the stem cell infusion. And her father reported an unexpected side effect: his libido was back. "That's just two people who were like, 'I don't even want to come to Rythmia.'" Alana said there's a vast number of conditions that can be healed through stem cell therapy, including, possibly, cancer. "We don't want to claim that it cures cancer," she said. "But you know, it could help."

But Alana said stem cell therapy was also a worthwhile investment for people who don't have any physical ailments, calling it preventative in addition to curative. And she appealed to our vanity. "Within twenty-four hours, you'll be able to feel and act younger." Doing the treatment at the end of an ayahuasca marathon was ideal, well worth the price, which ranged from $9,800 to $17,800, depending on whether you wanted ten million or fifty million pristine umbilical cord stem cells. "Ayahuasca is going to heal your past, and stem cells are going to turbocharge your future," she promised.

I asked Alana if she had peer-reviewed studies that backed up her claims. She said she did and promised to send me some by email. She followed up with a message that included links to three YouTube videos about stem cell research that were neither peer reviewed nor a validation of the pseudoscience on offer at Rythmia. The email said reported benefits from the therapy included higher zest for life and sex drive, increased muscle tone and bone density, improved cognitive function, smoother skin that is collagen- and elastin-rich, and the ability to "recover from strain and stress like a young person."

After the session, I did a Google search on stem cell therapy in Costa Rica and found that the country's medical association had issued a statement in 2018 warning of businesses that sell the useless and exorbitantly priced therapies to foreigners. In the United States, the FDA and the Federal Trade Commission have issued multiple warnings about the flourishing stem cell therapy marketplace, which has become a big business in the United States and in popular destinations for medical tourism, including Costa Rica and Panama.

I ran the claims from the session by Dr. Paul Knoepfler, a professor of cell biology at the University of California, Davis, who has become something of a watchdog in the booming industry of unregulated stem cell therapy. He told me that stem cell replacement therapy has only a few scientifically validated uses, to treat some blood and immune system disorders and certain cancers. But the type of infusion on offer at Rythmia, he said, was at best a prohibitively expensive placebo because the body usually attacks and kills foreign cells. In researching unscrupulous centers that offer miracle stem cell therapies, he has been struck by how gullible even well-educated people become when they're in distress. "There is this profound unhappiness with the current state of medicine, and people who are desperate are willing to roll the dice," he said. "In this case, throw in some sleep deprivation and psychedelics, and that will make people more highly suggestible."

A handful of Rythmia guests who had medical training rolled their eyes at the presentation and dismissed it as scammy. But I was struck by the fact that it didn't give them pause about the broader enterprise and messaging, which taps into people's frustration with and mistrust of the mainstream health care system. Quite a few of the guests during my week were psychotherapists who told me they had been drawn to Rythmia because they felt stuck in their profession and had lost faith in the tools at their disposal. One was an Australian woman who worked as a therapist at a large police department. She had decided to spend a whole month at Rythmia, which she called her "soul tribe." David, a therapist from Oregon, said that his time at Rythmia had been more cathartic and clarifying than the decades he spent in therapy. Then there was Hector, a psychologist from San Diego who had spent several years working for the federal government counseling Drug Enforcement Administration agents. They were thoughtful people, and I struggled to understand how they had fallen under the spell of Rythmia so easily, obediently swiping their wristbands each time they checked in for their colon cleanse and yoga class, and nodding along to the gospel of prosperity psychobabble we were power-washed with twenty hours a day. I asked questions, eager to understand how smart people can slip into a rabbit hole like this.

But on Wednesday, something unexpected happened. After my first Dead Sea Cleanse—which involved lying in a shallow tub as a small hose rinsed out my intestinal tract for thirty minutes—I felt a joyous sense of levity. In the afternoon, I went to the spa area, where I got a mud bath and then bounced back and forth between the cold plunge and the hot tub. I was surrounded by laughter and camaraderie as the time for the third ceremony neared. I found myself questioning whether I was being too dogmatic in my quest to find fault with the Rythmia way. The people around me all seemed to be having a blast, connecting with an intimacy that is rare in conventional interactions with strangers and drawing strength from each other as we put our bodies and minds through a punishing regimen.

Perhaps it was time for me to loosen my skepticism and see what happened to those who trust the process. There was heady anticipation about the ceremony that would begin in a few hours, an all-night raucous affair led by Taita Juanito, a Colombian *ayahuasquero* from the Ingano Indigenous community who has a devoted following among Rythmia regulars. Devotees say that drinking the powerful, sludge-like brew of ayahuasca that Taita Juanito brings from the Colombian state of Putumayo is entering the big leagues. Rythmia hypes Taita Juanito—whose name is Juan Guillermo Chindoy—describing him as a prodigy, a Doogie Howser of the shamanic world who was anointed as a Taita, or plant medicine elder, when he was a teenager. I had made small talk with Taita Juanito earlier in the week but struggled to make sense of anything that came out of his mouth. He has long, unkempt hair, a slight frame, and is prone to fits of giggles, which made him come across as more of a hippie than a guru.

By the time I walked up to him, shot glass in hand, my distrust had softened and my cynicism about Rythmia began giving way to a slight but certain doubt that I had been depriving myself of experiencing a miracle. People made impassioned, often tearful declarations about the dead relatives they had made peace with. A Black math teacher spoke movingly about connecting with enslaved ancestors. For others, the miracles were simple realizations, like discovering just how hard they had been on themselves. An hour into downing my cup, the familiar churning in my stomach began, my vision became blurry, and the silence in the room was interrupted by low grunts and heavy sighs. Suddenly, a string of words formed in my mind, taking me by surprise, giving way to an internal dialogue that happens often during ayahuasca sessions and feels quite distinct from the kind of rumination that normally unfolds in the mind.

I am ready for my miracle, I found myself declaring silently.

Make a wish, the response came.

My answer was unexpected but resolute, as though I had been suppressing a deeply held desire that had finally been uncorked: *I want to see my grandmother Natalia*, I said silently. I was momentarily startled by the request and its earnestness, because, in the moment, I believed she could somehow be summoned from the place where the souls of dead people linger. In the weeks prior to coming to Rythmia, I had spent a lot of time trying to piece together the history of mental illness in the family. The endeavor had left me feeling that I had only scratched the surface with Natalia. I longed to find out how she ended up undergoing electroshock therapy for depression, whether it helped, and how she became such a fervent disciple of Freudian psychoanalysis, which she had imposed on my father. Suddenly, it seemed possible that I could ask her questions, pin her down on details, join her in the realm of the dead, or bring her momentarily to the land of the living on this blue planet spinning in the dark. But more than that, I wanted to feel the warmth and love of a woman who looked so sullen and withdrawn in the black-and-white portraits that had provided my only glimpse into her life. I wanted to hold her and to be held and walk away convinced that there was a wise elder looking out for me from the beyond.

The room was heady with fragrant smoke that a woman fanned out from a pot. The din of vomiting, moans, and laughter that had filled the silence during the first couple of hours of the ceremony was drowned out by drums that were the centerpiece of a frenetic set of music.

Don't think, drink. The words that had felt so reckless and insane just days ago now taunted me and propelled me to push my woozy body off the mat and stagger toward Taita, shot glass in hand. Before handing me a new serving, Taita blew into the glass, making a dramatic whoosh sound. Soon I was reaching for a third gulp in order to lean, ever more doggedly, into the fantasy that a portal to Natalia was within reach. *Don't drink, think.* As the third cup began seeping into my bloodstream, my ability to form cogent thoughts frayed, and for a moment, I was enticed by the possibility that it heralded a breakthrough. But it led merely to a blackout.

Birds were chirping, and dawn had broken when I got my bearings again. There was a pungent smell in the air, and I soon spotted the source: soiled mattresses had been laid out a few feet from my mat. I noticed a woman sitting cross-legged on her mat, weeping. Soon, we were summoned to gather at the center of the room, where Taita held court. He talked about the creation of the universe, spirits, the natural world, and love, the wonder of love, in a jumble of sentences that lacked connective tissue and a discernible takeaway. When Taita stopped speaking, a handful of participants delivered grandiose I-had-my-miracle speeches. It took conscious effort not to roll my eyes, and yet I was torn between jealousy for the feelings of release and catharsis on display and of deep shame for how close I had come the night before to falling into the Rythmia trance. My skepticism roared back that morning as we were subjected to a new marketing pitch, this time for the Rythmia aftercare program—online offerings including yoga, breath work, and meditation—for a $999 fee. Those who had not quite gotten their miracle were encouraged to put down a $500 deposit to lock in the current rates and come back to Rythmia to try again. Then came the most astounding upsell: those truly committed to the Rythmia way could spend $710,000 to become among the inaugural homeowners in "the best spiritual community on the planet." That would be Rythmia Residences, a fifty-acre, one-hundred-unit residential compound under construction near the resort, where the $1,100 monthly HOA fees would include ayahuasca ceremonies and breath work sessions.

〰 I saw Gerry for the first time midweek at lunchtime. He was sitting at Roots, Rythmia's restaurant, by himself. I introduced myself and mentioned that I was a journalist working on a book about medicinal psychedelics. I had been transparent about this when I booked my slot in April, and I wondered whether there would be any effort to set ground rules regarding what I could and couldn't report on, or whether I would be given VIP treatment. Neither happened. Gerry was charming and warm and said he would be delighted to sit down for an interview toward the end of the week. For now, he counseled, I should focus on drinking as much ayahuasca as humanly possible, to lose myself during the ceremonies that remained. *Drink, don't think.*

At the end of the week, when we sat down to talk, I steeled myself for an adversarial interview. It was hard to know where to start given how many disturbing things I had seen over the course of the week. But as we spoke, a stream of outgoing guests stopped by to thank Gerry effusively. A gray-haired nurse who had come with her son, a Rythmia frequent flier, called it "the best week of my life." A schoolteacher who had recently left her husband after he was charged with a sexual crime involving a minor told him she "was going home whole."

So I found myself asking Gerry gentler questions than I had intended. I asked him how the clientele had changed since they first opened in 2015. He said they used to get mainly hippies, "searchers that didn't have a history of success in their lives." But over time, Rythmia started attracting "super-successful people," which he prefers, because they tend to have more radical transformations under the influence of ayahuasca than people who have been on a spiritual path for years. I told him I had found the sleep deprivation regimen disorienting and taxing. Gerry smiled. It was by design, he said. "The more worn down they are, the more their ego sits down." I noted that it also made people suggestible and asked about the propriety of bombarding people with offers to buy more products and services. Gerry chuckled, and his candor surprised me. "We try to give you every chance to part with your money," he said, arguing that money spent at Rythmia is money well spent. "Of all the things people could spend money on, it's probably the least harmful thing they could ever spend money on in their lives."

I asked him how he thought about cultural appropriation, as he was one of the leading figures taking Amazonian traditions and imbuing them with a prosperity ethos along with other twists, like the colonics. Gerry said that keeping traditions static amounts to giving in to "peer pressure from dead people." It's up to those of us now alive to collectively decide which parts of ancient traditions to preserve and which to ditch and to embrace the blending of traditions.

I asked him how much work he still had to do to heal. "A ton," he said without hesitation. His biggest struggle was laziness, which he said ayahuasca is constantly chiding him for. "I'm lazier than she wants me to be," he said. "She's unrelenting. She just keeps asking me for more, more, more, more."

To what end? I asked. "To balance out what's going on." As in to balance out all the ills of the world? I asked mockingly. He responded matter-of-factly: "I believe so."

I wondered whether Gerry believed—*truly* believed—the story at the heart of his miracle, if he had absolute certainty that his grandfather had been a pedophile. Gerry's response surprised me. The truth was immaterial, he argued. "Whether you're remembering the way that you felt about it or whether it actually happened, it's the same thing."

Before wrapping up, I told Gerry I was having trouble with the whole miracle trope. Clearly, it worked for many people, giving them a sense that they had been touched by magic, rescued by divine forces. But it seemed to set the bar too high, to push people to delude themselves, and to what end, exactly? Gerry was animated by the question. The goal, he said, is to awaken people to all the wonder and mystery of being alive, to remind people how weird and extraordinary it is that we're all sharing this planet, to open people's eyes to the tiny and gigantic mysteries of existence. "That bird that just flew there," he said, pointing toward the pool. "Tell me how that happens? Tell me how that fucking happens."

There's a graduation ritual on the final day of a Rythmia week, during which the final miracle reports are shared and the staff pleads with guests who had an amazing experience to leave a detailed review on TripAdvisor. There was a final plug for the aftercare program and a reminder that outgoing guests who want to return should put down a deposit before leaving campus. Then, without warning, little aquamarine cards were passed out, and Bernie, the former car executive, asked us to stand up. The card contained the Rythmia Oath. I stood in stunned silence as the vast majority of those around me recited it with conviction:

> *I (first and last name), hereby pledge in front of you, my brothers and sisters, that something in me has completed. I have reached a point of freedom and it is my intention to maintain this freedom. I am now one with my soul and ready to participate more fully in the world than I ever have before. My obligation to you, and all living beings, is simply to keep this connection with myself clear and clean. I intend to maintain my spiritual practice so that this can occur. I can fulfill my destiny as a light worker–warrior. I promise I will fully practice in this gift of life by touching those who I encounter with my merged soul. By doing this together, we become the living shift. This is my agreement to you.*

As if reading my mind, Bernie said, "Remember, we're not a cult, we're a club."

Rythmia Postscript

After leaving Rythmia, I wanted to dig a bit deeper into the history of this not-cult. It was clear to me that many of the guests chose Rythmia, buying into its promise to serve ayahuasca in a safe, luxurious, and "medically licensed" establishment. But I soon found that key parts of its origin story and its claim to have a medical license are deeply misleading.

When Rythmia formally launched in February 2015, it announced in a press release that it would offer a novel form of "addiction rehabilitation" that it had previously made available to "the rich and famous." The key ingredient was iboga, the African plant that was

Gerry's introduction to psychedelics, and his shaman, Moughenda, was a partner in the venture. The press release offered something virtually no other rehab does: "a MONEY-BACK GUARANTEE."

But Moughenda's tenure at Rythmia was short. In March 2015, law enforcement officials in Costa Rica were trying to find Moughenda after a Norwegian woman who sought treatment for addiction died in his care, according to press reports. Dr. Allan Varela, a senior official at Costa Rica's health ministry, said his team opened an investigation into Rythmia's operations and soon learned that Moughenda had fled the country. Allan said Rythmia ceased using iboga and told health officials it would only treat patients with a fasting protocol. But soon it simply switched to ayahuasca. By importing and commercializing the brew, Allan said, Rythmia and retreat centers like it are breaking drug laws. But because Costa Rica decriminalized personal use of controlled substances, tourists who participate in retreats are in the clear. The government has turned a blind eye to this booming trade, Allan added, because it has become an increasingly larger share of the tourism market. "The great majority of the people who go to them are foreigners," he said. "Perhaps that's why we seldom get complaints."

But complaints about Rythmia have been growing among former employees and guests. I tracked down a former Rythmia yoga teacher, Candice-Marie Fox, who said she was fired in 2019 after confronting Gerry and his leadership team about practices she found exploitative and unethical. The staff, she said, were trained to coax guests into believing they had attained a miracle, often making a big deal out of flimsy or vague insights or sensations they had experienced during ceremonies. Then, at the peak of their sleeplessness, she said, the sales team would pounce. "You would be hunting them down, finding someone to sell to," said Candice-Marie, who was initially hired as a yoga teacher in 2017, and spent roughly two years working at Rythmia. Unbeknownst to guests, staffers earned a commission on sales and competed ruthlessly to go after customers who appeared amenable to buying stem cells, the aftercare package, or an upcoming week. "It was dog-eat-dog," she said.

Candice-Marie said that the majority of guests leave feeling healed and energized, believing they had experienced something miraculous. But she came to think of the process as a form of groupthink that gave many people a short-lived sense of transformation. There was a script for the small number of guests who neared the end of the week feeling miracle-deprived. "The way we used to gaslight them was by saying, 'Your expectations are too high. You need to drink more,'" she told me.

That's what happened to Jenna Williams, an Arizona woman who makes a living bagging groceries at a supermarket to support herself and a daughter. She had first heard about Rythmia watching a video posted by Kyle Cease, a comedian and author who was invited to attend the retreat as a speaker. "The people who run it are amazing people with huge hearts on a mission to make you feel better," he gushed in one of several videos he recorded recommending the resort. "As the week goes by, you start feeling softer, you start breathing again, and it's not even expensive here. For what they're giving you, it's ridiculously affordable."

Soon, Jenna spotted a magazine article on sale at her cashier station featuring Lindsay Lohan's ayahuasca experience. "She said she had found her purpose, and that's what clicked for me," she said. "I wanted to find my purpose."

The cost was prohibitive for her, but Jenna took a leap of faith, signed up for a week in February 2018, and put it on a credit card. By the end of the week, she felt severely anxious and disappointed by all the miracle tales the other guests were telling. "I felt like I didn't surrender enough to the medicine," she said. A Rythmia employee suggested she stay an additional week to try anew, but Jenna needed to return home to take care of her daughter. But she was persuaded to purchase the aftercare program and to leave a deposit for another visit. She returned in August, determined to attend all the sessions and to more fully trust the process. She barely slept all week and ate little. The day of her departure, Jenna said, her thinking became paranoid and delusional; she felt terrified of leaving Rythmia. She fell to the ground near the pool, screaming as the new guests were streaming in. Rythmia staff whisked her out of sight. Over the next few days, she was confined in a small room in the clinic as the staff forced her to take medicine that put her to sleep, sometimes forcibly squirting something into her mouth with a syringe. "I felt very childlike," she said. "Nothing was explained to me."

Roughly five days after Jenna had been scheduled to return home, Rythmia got in touch with the friend listed as an emergency contact. Soon, her mother was on a plane to Costa Rica, where Jeff McNairy, Rythmia's chief medical officer, told her Jenna's case was not an aberration. "He told her that this happens all the time, that it takes longer for some people to come out of it than others," Jenna said. She was sent home and instructed to continue taking Rispolux, a drug used to treat schizophrenia and psychotic episodes. Her mood stabilized after she returned to Arizona, but the debt she had taken on to pay for her time at Rythmia forced her to take two additional jobs. In addition to her supermarket job, she took shifts delivering goods through Amazon Flex and Instacart. But it wasn't enough; she filed for bankruptcy during the pandemic. "I was working myself literally to death doing three jobs and school and raising my daughter," she said.

Soon after getting in touch with Jenna, I heard from Zinlynn Somerville, a paralegal in Canada who wanted to tell me her own Rythmia nightmare story. Zinlynn had first traveled to Costa Rica in August 2018 to drink ayahuasca at the suggestion of her therapist, who tagged along for the journey. Early in the week, Gerry showered her with attention and told her he had had a dream about her, said Zinlynn, who initially found the remark creepy but inconsequential. After she checked out, she said she was feeling dazed and struggled to make sense of the experience when Gerry sent her a message on Facebook and urged her to come back. When she did, in April 2019, she said Gerry summoned her to his hotel room to share an important announcement. "The medicine has been telling me for months,

'Don't worry, the love of your life is coming,'" Zinlynn remembers Gerry telling her. The moon, Gerry said, had been quite specific, saying his beloved was an Asian woman with two children. "We need to explore this," Zinlynn remembered hearing from him. "We have to listen to the medicine. If you don't listen to the medicine, you're not going to live your best life."

Zinlynn said she found Gerry unattractive, but she was flattered by his interest and found the idea that their romance was preordained alluring. They weren't physically intimate that week, but Gerry persuaded her to fly back soon. Zinlynn checked into a nearby hotel, to have autonomy in case their initial date didn't go well. Gerry showed up with San Pedro, a psychedelic derived from a cactus, and told her she needed to drink it to balance her masculine and feminine energies. Zinlynn said the two had sex that night under the influence of drugs.

After that visit, Gerry told her to move down to Rythmia permanently. She was smitten and eager to quit her job. By December 2019, she was living at Rythmia. "I thought, *This is a changed man who is healing people*," Zinlynn said. "*And law is so boring.*"

There was no honeymoon period. Behind closed doors, she said, Gerry drank heavily, smoked, and began treating her with disdain. "He started abusing me, calling me names," she said. His mood darkened when Rythmia shut down during the pandemic, she added, and one night, in a drunken rage, Gerry slapped her across the face. "In the morning, he apologized to me profusely, and then he recorded a video saying that the reason he had to hit me was that I was possessed by the devil," she said. The remedy was to drink more ayahuasca, Gerry told her. Their relationship unraveled when Zinlynn had what she described as a psychotic break one night when, under the influence of ayahuasca, she had visions of Gerry shooting her. She announced the next day that she was leaving, but was kept there against her will for six days, Zinlynn said. When she was finally allowed to leave, Zinlynn said, she was handed a nondisclosure agreement offering to pay her $30,000 in exchange for a vow not to discuss her time at Rythmia publicly. Zinlynn said she refused, believing she had a duty to warn others about a place she came to see as a cult. After leaving Rythmia for good, she's struggled to make sense of how she ignored all the red flags, she said. Her conclusion: it's surprisingly easy to fall under the spell of a narcissist. "I believe Gerry thinks God chose him to do this work," she said. "And a lot of people worship him."

3

~~~~~~~~~

IN CHURCHES AND CLINICS, AMERICANS TURN TO PSYCHEDELICS TO HEAL

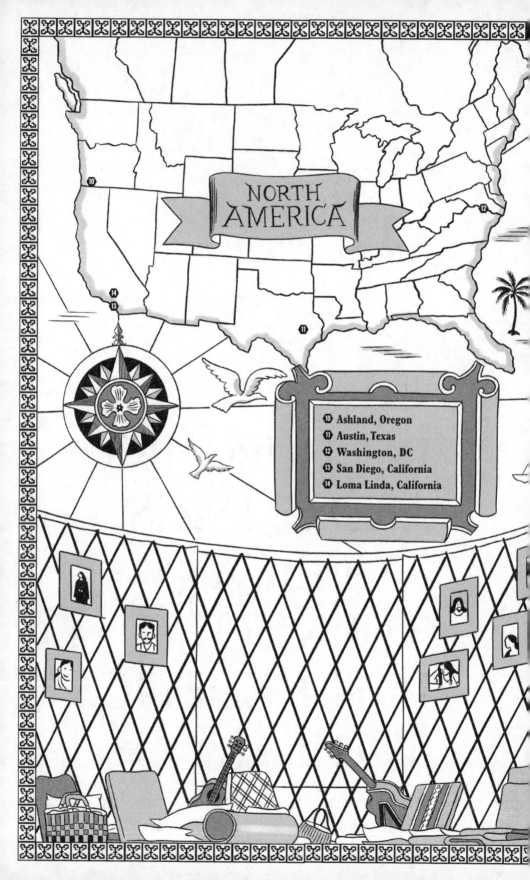

NORTH AMERICA

10 Ashland, Oregon
11 Austin, Texas
12 Washington, DC
13 San Diego, California
14 Loma Linda, California

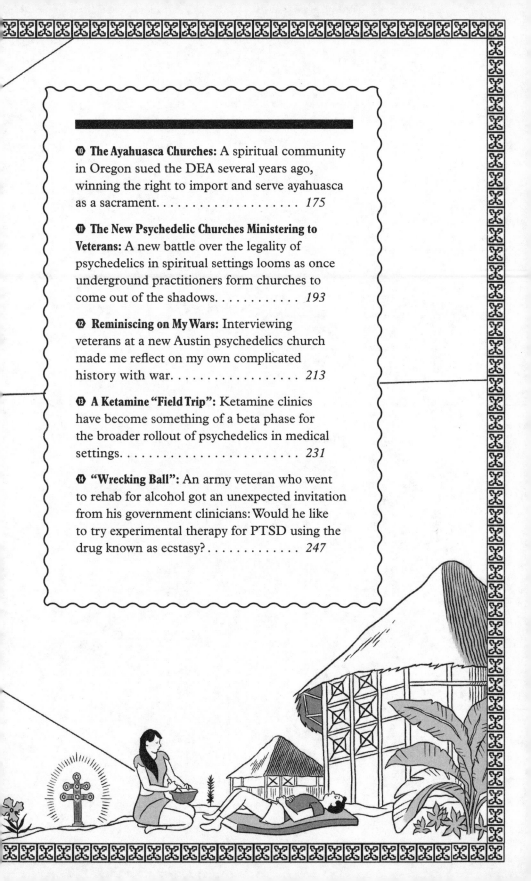

10 THE AYAHUASCA CHURCHES

SURELY THE DRIVER HAD MADE a wrong turn, Aaron Goldman thought as he watched a large RV lumber up the unpaved road that leads to his family home in a bucolic spot in southern Oregon.

"I'm getting ready to walk outside and be like, 'Hey, you're in the wrong place. Can I help you find where you're trying to go?'" Aaron recalled, when the vehicle pulled up, federal law enforcement officers in bulletproof vests burst out, and barged inside the home, pointing weapons at Aaron, who was then sixteen, and at his younger sister, Zara, then fourteen. It was May 1999, and his family was the latest target of the war on drugs.

Acting on a tip, agents from the Drug Enforcement Administration were looking for jugs of ayahuasca that Aaron's parents, Jonathan and Jane, had smuggled from Brazil. The couple had been serving the brew for years at clandestine services of the Church of the Holy Light of the Queen, which they founded in 1996 after becoming initiates of Santo Daime, the syncretic Christian religion founded in the early twentieth century by rubber tappers in the Brazilian Amazon.

Aaron's parents were away. As the agents rummaged through the home, they barraged him with questions about his parents' spiritual practice: Did kids attend services? Had Jonathan and Jane forced their children to drink the bitter-tasting tea?

"These two guys were totally doing the good cop, bad cop thing," Aaron said. "One was trying to be our friend, while the other guy is saying that we're never going to see our parents again."

That morning, Jonathan and Jane had driven to the home of a congregant who had just passed away from complications of AIDS. They comforted the relatives sitting by the man's bed, where he had been lying wearing the *farda*, or uniform, Santo Daime initiates wear.

Sitting by the corpse had been a "beautiful moment of peace," Jonathan told me. Their solemn, reflective mood was shattered as the couple pulled into their driveway and found the large RV. Moments after he stepped out of the car, agents put Jonathan in handcuffs and took him to jail. In addition to the freshly arrived containers of ayahuasca, investigators seized computers, documents, and other evidence. Jane was not taken into custody.

"They had an expectation that they were going to find a drug dealer and that this was a new drug imported from South America," Jonathan recalled, chuckling. "They thought they were going to find, you know, pornography and guns and people lying around, shooting up, that kind of thing."

Instead, he said, the agents stumbled into a cozy, well-appointed home with "crystals and pictures of saints, and they didn't know what to do."

The raid by DEA agents was the opening salvo of a legal fight at the intersection of counternarcotics policy and religious freedom laws that dragged on for roughly a decade. It was set in motion by simultaneous raids on two American affiliates of Brazilian churches that use ayahuasca as sacraments. As DEA agents raided the Goldman home, another team searched the New Mexico offices of Jeffrey Bronfman, the American leader of União do Vegetal, a spiritist

Christian church that had also been importing ayahuasca illegally to administer as a sacrament.

After reviewing the evidence collected during the searches, federal prosecutors in Oregon and New Mexico opted not to charge Goldman and Bronfman with drug crimes. This was notable. There was no doubt both men had been importing and administering a drink that contains N-dimethyltryptamine, or DMT, which the federal government has labeled as a dangerous drug with no known medical value. But prosecutors made clear their decision to not pursue criminal cases should not be interpreted as tacit permission to keep the churches open, Jonathan said. The top federal prosecutor in Oregon, he told me, conveyed to Jonathan's lawyer: "If I ever hear that Mr. Goldman is importing that tea or doing rituals, I'm going to come and get him."

Besides the threat of criminal prosecution, the Goldmans had also risked losing custody of their children. Child protection services officials interviewed Aaron and Zara at their school about their parents as the government contemplated whether they should be put in foster care, Jane told me. "That was really scary, that was the scariest thing for the kids and for us."

I asked Jonathan whether the lingering threat of prosecution and the trauma inflicted on their children made them question their faith in Santo Daime. Quite the opposite, he told me. "When we started in the Daime, we knew a day like this was going to come," he said. "We knew the day of confrontation with the government was going to come somehow, someway."

〰〰 Having missed their chance to fight the government as defendants, Jonathan and Jeffrey went on the offensive: they sued the government. The two men had escaped prosecution, but neither intended to stop ministering to their communities, which meant continuing to operate under a shadow of illegality. The only way to change that was by taking a swipe at the Controlled Substances Act, which has remained the backbone of the war on drugs since it was passed in 1970 during the Nixon administration. The ayahuasca churches would seek to persuade federal judges that prohibition was an affront to their religious freedoms. The lawsuits raised eyebrows at the Department of Justice, where officials were wary of being dragged into a case at the intersection of drug policy and religious freedoms.

"It was a bold move," Liza Goitein, who was then a trial attorney at the Department of Justice assigned to defend the lawsuit brought by União do Vegetal. "Rather than being happy to have escaped prosecution, they were going to poke the bear."

At the time, there was little legal precedent on the sacramental use of compounds that are illegal and classified as dangerous drugs. The limited guidance that existed pertained to the use of peyote, a psychoactive cactus, in Native American Church rituals.

In 1981, Theodore Olson, who was then the assistant attorney general in charge of the Office of Legal Counsel, issued a memorandum to the DEA asserting that the use of peyote in NAC rituals should be regarded as permissible use of a sacrament. Citing the church's long-standing use of peyote, and the central role it plays in the community's cosmology, Olson argued it warranted a narrow dispensation under the Controlled Substances Act. "As a practical matter, we believe that no religion other than the NAC would qualify for the exemption," he wrote.

The carve-out applied only to federal law, which set the stage for a legal dispute that reached the Supreme Court in 1990. It involved two members of the Native American Church, coincidentally from Oregon, who were fired from a private drug rehabilitation clinic and denied unemployment benefits over their use of peyote. The Supreme Court sided with Oregon, finding that the state's prohibition of peyote was reasonable and constitutional because it applied to all people and did not single out members of a faith community.

The ruling riled up religious freedom groups, which lobbied Congress to enact broader protections, citing concerns that the ruling could undermine religious freedoms in a wide range of scenarios, including health care services, zoning rules, and building ordinances. Heeding their call, in 1993, Congress set a higher bar for the state to restrict the activities of religious groups by passing the Religious Freedom Restoration Act. During a bill-signing ceremony, President Bill Clinton hailed the law, saying the government should be held "to a very high level of proof before it interferes with someone's free exercise of religion." Under the law, the government may meddle in the affairs of a church "only in furtherance of a compelling government interest." And it can only apply the "least restrictive means" to advance that goal.

The following year, Congress passed another law that barred states from prohibiting the use of peyote by members of the NAC.

A little over a year after the ayahuasca church raids, Jeffrey, a member of a wealthy Canadian family that traces its fortune to a bootlegging operation during Prohibition, hired an experienced team of lawyers in a quest to legalize the sacramental use of ayahuasca. In its complaint, the church stated that drinking ayahuasca was a "central and essential tenet" of the church and that members regarded the tea as "a manifestation of Divinity."

The União do Vegetal and Santo Daime cases presented a dilemma for the government because religious freedom law did not provide a process for the government to consider or implement the kind of administrative exemptions the plaintiffs were seeking, Liza told me. "I think the government finds it both as a matter of principle and as a matter of politics very problematic to be weighing in on what should be deemed a legitimate religion," Liza said.

Ultimately, the DEA mounted a vigorous defense, arguing that loopholes and exemptions would undermine their enforcement system, she said. Justice Department attorneys conceded that seizing shipments of ayahuasca burdened the free exercise of UDV members, but argued that the ban was necessary to protect the health of church members, to prevent the diversion of the tea to recreational users, and to comply with a 1971 United Nations convention on drugs.

〰〰 The case made it to the Supreme Court, which, in February 2006, issued a unanimous ruling in favor of the UDV, forcing the DEA to establish a mechanism for church leaders to import their tea lawfully.

Seeking to attain the same benefit, Jonathan Goldman filed a similar lawsuit in Oregon, arguing that confiscating their tea amounted to treating Christ as contraband. "The Holy Daime tea is believed to be not only a vehicle for direct communion with God, but itself embodies the Divine Spirit," the complaint says. "According to Church doctrine, the presence of the Daime is the presence of Christ."

Jonathan crackled with enthusiasm as he recalled the trial before Judge Owen M. Panner, an octogenarian who became fascinated by the history of Santo Daime. When a government lawyer suggested one of the hymns condoned the use of marijuana, church members pushed back and asked if they could sing a few bars to show the judge how beautiful and profound the song was. "I loved being on the stand," Jonathan told me. "I had been rehearsing for ten years in the shower, if you know what I mean, wondering what they were going to ask me."

In a twenty-two-page ruling, Judge Panner provided a strikingly detailed history of Santo Daime and its rituals. "As the Daime tea takes effect, members may sit quietly with eyes half-closed," the judge wrote. "Users describe the experience as dream-like. They may experience visual effects, although not true hallucinations (i.e. the person is aware that the effect is not real); alterations in the perception of time and space; and intense emotions, including euphoria. Users report profound insights into their personal problems."

Panner found that the government had failed to prove that "outright prohibition" of the tea was the "least restrictive means of furthering its interests." He also concluded that the plaintiffs had "established that they are sincere in their religious beliefs, and that the ceremonial use of the Daime tea is essential to their religion."

The ruling forced the DEA, which had been deeply reluctant to broaden the range of religious practitioners authorized to use psychedelics, to establish an exemption and regulatory system for churches.

〰 Jonathan's spiritual awakening was set in motion when he was in his early twenties. Around then, Jonathan told me, he began hearing a voice in his head that appeared to emanate from another realm, like a radio that suddenly starts picking a new signal. Since then, he has come to believe that every step of his journey as a healer and spiritual leader has been guided by spiritual entities that long ago identified him as a medium and have been propelling him forward, often in directions that felt uncomfortable and daunting at the time.

He trained as an acupuncturist at a time when the Chinese medicine modality was virtually unknown in the West and later became a disciple of bioenergetics, a form of psychotherapy that relies on movement, breathing techniques, and other tools to dissolve trauma and stress. Jonathan studied bioenergetics under José Rosa, a Portuguese-born therapist who spent much of his adult life in Brazil before moving to the Boston area.

In 1987, José told Jonathan that he was going to take him to a place in the mountains in Brazil, where they would spend a month doing "the equivalent of ten years of meditation and ten years of therapy," Jonathan told me. He was given few details. His introduction to Santo Daime was mind-blowing. "I was like an envelope that someone turned inside out," he told me. Everything he had come to understand about healing seemed like child's play. "I felt like I was a YMCA basketball player and, you know, I was really good, and one day I go to the gym and Michael Jordan shows up."

A few months after his initiation, Jonathan returned to Brazil with José and traveled to a Santo Daime enclave in the Amazon jungle called Céu do Mapiá, where they spent a month. Jonathan had two young children at home, and Jane was growing resentful of the time and money he was devoting to this strange newfound passion. But there was no turning back, he told me.

Six months later, he returned to Brazil to become a *fardado*, a uniform-wearing initiate. Over the next three years, Jonathan brought Americans down to Brazil for monthlong workshops to introduce them to Santo Daime. Jane, who was initially skeptical of a religion that required learning Portuguese and wearing a formal uniform, eventually fell in love with Santo Daime as well. It happened, she told me, when she had a *miração* that showed her a path to keep her family united in love.

In the early 1990s, Alex Polari, the Santo Daime elder, who had become a close friend and mentor to Jonathan, asked him whether he was interested in opening a church in the United States. Jonathan demurred.

"I'm not getting any divine messages," Jonathan told Alex.

"Another one who wants to hear Gabriel's trumpet!" Alex replied with a chuckle.

"What's wrong with that?" Jonathan asked.

"There's nothing wrong with that. That's just not how it works most of the time," Alex said.

But soon, Jonathan began packing bottles of ayahuasca in his carry-on bags as he prepared to return to the United States. He and Jane started leading Santo Daime services in Oregon for a tiny community of initiates who had gotten their start in Brazil. Over the years, the community grew to a few dozen members, but it has remained small and low profile. Newcomers find the church through word of mouth, and core members adhere to the religion's strict rule against proselytizing. "I came from the leftist American political movement, and we were always proselytizing," Jonathan told me, referring to the counterculture movement in the 1970s. "So it was a great relief to just do the work."

Early in life, both of their children resented how much time and energy their parents devoted to the church, they told me. But as adults, they independently gravitated toward Santo Daime and became *fardados*.

At the end of our conversation, Jonathan suggested I consider attending one of the church's "self-transformation workshops," a three-day program the Goldmans hold a handful of times per year for people who are curious about Santo Daime. The idea of drinking ayahuasca in the United States in the rare place where doing so is entirely legal was appealing. Doing so under the tutelage of a formerly Jewish family that now sings devotional songs to Jesus and the Virgin Mary—not so much. Though I was raised by parents who were not particularly devout Catholics, I dutifully underwent the rites of passage—baptism, First Communion, and confirmation—and the church's homophobia had made me feel like a sinner and an outcast. I wasn't eager to reconnect to any aspect of Catholicism, even through a three-day ayahuasca workshop.

〰 As I pondered Jonathan's workshop invitation, I picked up his book, which was published in 2014. Jonathan posits that each person is a soul that gets deposited on earth for a learning experience that is shaped by past lives, or our karma. Suffering, he writes, is a means to learn the lessons we are meant to learn in each lifetime. And the only way to lessen our "karmic imprint" is to master the hard but indispensable act of forgiveness—by learning to forgive ourselves and others.

I was intrigued by Jonathan's theory. Here was a secular Jew who became the American leader of a Brazilian syncretic Christian religion, and yet his belief system seemed to borrow heavily from Buddhism. To boot, he was a self-professed medium who had beaten the DEA in court.

The first step to securing a spot at an upcoming "self-transformation workshop," which cost $950, was filling out a lengthy questionnaire that covered my basic medical history and posed a few odd questions. "What are your main talents, skills and accomplishments?" the church wanted to know. Also: "Have you experienced any of the following: spiritual awakening or emergency? A psychic experience?"

What the hell is a spiritual emergency? I wondered. I checked *no* on the psychic experience.

After the church team that screens new members reviewed my application, I got a call from Mona Tara, an internal medicine physician and veteran church member. Her hour-long calls are designed to make sure prospective workshop attendants know what to expect. I instantly liked Mona. She was warm, funny, and down to earth. When I told her about my aversion to Christian symbols, she confided they had been a struggle for her when she first drifted into Santo Daime. Two things stood out from our conversation. She told me that unlike most mainstream ayahuasca centers and retreats, the church does not disqualify people who are taking antidepressants and other psychiatric drugs, having concluded that there is no compelling scientific evidence that mixing the two is risky. Church leaders, she said, feel duty bound to help individuals who have complicated psychiatric histories, the kind of people who get excluded from psychedelic clinical studies and mainstream retreats.

Toward the end of our call, almost as an afterthought, Mona mentioned I would likely see mediumship in action. *Huh?* During services, she explained, some veteran church members serve as mediums for spiritual entities that have unfinished business on the terrestrial plane. This can look and sound disconcerting to newcomers, Mona allowed. But she asked me to try to avoid staring at mediums in a trance or to focus too much on the whole thing. It's just a thing that happens in Daime circles, she said, and she didn't want it to catch me off guard.

〰〰 I arrived at Jonathan and Jane's home, where the church is located, on a crisp, cloudless Thursday morning. As instructed, I was dressed in white, a requirement for Daime ceremonies, which are called *trabalhos*, or works, because, as Daimistas are prone to remind newcomers, they are often laborious and draining sessions. In fact, Jonathan told us, every single Daimista initiate has experienced two things: a moment where "you swear you will never drink another cup," and a rough *trabalho* during which "you think you're dying—and not metaphorically."

The *trabalhos* in Ashland are held in a pair of yurts shrouded by imposing pine trees. The smaller yurt contains an altar where the Daime is served in small shot glasses. Participants form two lines, segregated by gender, to take the sacrament. Then each person sits in a designated spot inside the larger yurt, which is also segregated by gender. In the middle of the room, there is an altar with a two-barred cross, a bowl of water, a candle, and a vase with freshly cut flowers.

The cross is placed strategically in the middle of the yurt, just below a skylight cone that lets light stream in. The opening serves as a conduit for spiritual entities to descend into the ceremony room, church leaders explained. It also can be used as a channel to unburden ourselves of entities and energies that don't serve us, Jonathan said. "Put your prayers at the foot of the cross," he instructed. "All we let go of goes to the cosmic recycling center." The water bowl, we were told, symbolizes "the divine feminine." It represents the state of "flowing" and the beauty of tears. The candle is a symbol of "masculine energy," a reminder of the "principle of active transformation." The flowers, meanwhile, were an emblem of the process of "rebirth and renewal."

Jonathan informed the veteran churchgoers which hymnbooks they would be singing from. Newcomers were instructed to simply breathe and focus on the music and our shifting sensations, making a concerted effort to "open our hearts." Once the singing starts, the collective vibration in the room would rise, forming a "current of compassion." A chain of hearts would suddenly beat as one as we snapped into the same frequency. "Our hearts seek each other," Jonathan said. "Hearts seek hearts."

Before we got going, he urged us to check any and all expectations at the door. "There's a divine intelligence that will say: you need to do this, focus on that memory, that addiction, that trauma," he said. But the Daime acts autonomously with priorities and logic that are often befuddling. "It's not going to happen how you expect it," Jonathan said. "The Daime is much smarter than us—what a relief!"

ᄊᄊ My body recoiled as I gulped down the first glass of ayahuasca, which Daimistas call simply Daime. Most of my ayahuasca experience has been in pitch-dark settings, and there was something transfixing about feeling the brew kick in while sitting in a light-filled room.

As a Portuguese speaker, I was offered a hymnbook to follow along. When the music began, I was taken aback by the rigidity of the beat, which is punctuated by the synchronized shake of maracas wielded by experienced Daimistas. The singing felt militant, like a soundtrack for a marching band. Church members sang with stoicism in accented Portuguese. I found myself scanning the small, dog-eared hymnbook like a hawk, on alert for terms that triggered me. "*Soften the hearts of these sinful people*," they sang. Pleas were directed to "*the always Virgin Mary*" and to the "*divine baby Jesus.*"

Beyond the religious symbols, there seemed to be two dominant themes in the hymns. They call on Daimistas to pay attention, closely, to sharpen their ability to see and understand things clearly. "*Whoever is on this path, walk very slowly*," one of the songs commanded. "*Pay close attention, to avoid erring.*"

Several hymns exhort worshippers to cultivate *firmeza*, a term that means "a state of steadiness and resoluteness." Daimistas are taught to approach all the difficult aspects of life—including love, fear, and faith—with *firmeza*. The two bananas I had scarfed down that morning—the only food I would have for the day—churned audibly as a heavy feeling of nausea set in. But instead of contracting into a fetal position, like the guy next to me had, I steadied my back and kept my eyes locked on the prayer book, embracing *firmeza* as a challenge, a practice.

But soon, my attempt at steadfastness was derailed when I spotted Jonathan's daughter, Zara, start to shake as her face contorted into anguished expressions. Putting down her prayer book, Zara pushed herself off the ground and began walking unsteadily as her parents watched with a knowing smile. A spirit guide known as *Sete Flechas*, or Seven Arrows, had descended into the *trabalho*, we were later informed, and used Zara's body, as he often did, to impart some wisdom. In slurring Portuguese, Zara spoke about the futility of obsessive thinking. She spoke in hushed tones, which made it hard for me to follow much of what she said. "Nothing is guaranteed," she said. "But if you don't make an effort, for sure nothing will happen." After about five minutes, *Sete Flechas* appeared to exit, and Zara collapsed back in her seat, looking exhausted. My mind was left reeling.

Soon, it was happening again. Shannon Ransom, a woman with long white hair and sad blue eyes, began yelping as her shoulders jerked up and down. As she slipped into a trance, the singing got louder and faster, as though the volume was necessary to give Shannon strength. Mona's suggestion that we refrain from staring at mediums in action was useless. My eyes were glued on Shannon as she got up on her feet, her gaze darting wildly across the room, and staggered toward the altar, taking a knee just a couple of feet from me. Her spine moved in wavelike jolts as her hands thrust skyward. A couple of church veterans stood alongside Shannon, pointing their open palms toward her, like they were radiating support. After what felt like an eternity, Shannon's shaking ebbed, the music returned to a gentler tempo, and everyone kept singing as though nothing out of the ordinary had transpired.

Suddenly, Jonathan announced it was time for the third and final serving of Daime that day. Reading my mind, he said, "There will come a point when the time to drink Daime comes and you say, 'Heck no!'" But he urged us to override that reluctance. "Fear has no voice these days. There is nothing to be afraid of. The antidote to fear is faith."

〜〜〜 As I settled into bed on the first night, still feeling a slight buzz from the Daime, I was dazzled by what I had witnessed. I was convinced the mediumship episodes had not been an act. That left two options: I could take them at face value, allowing for the possibility that many of us unknowingly swim in a sea of tortured souls, invisible energetic beings that have the potential to uplift and torment us. Or I could dismiss these dramatic scenes as hallucinations, short-lasting psychotic breaks. But there was something notable about this church. Its leaders seemed unconcerned with whether those of us who were new to their rituals walked away as true believers. If this was a cult, or cult-adjacent, wouldn't there be more of an effort to convince us about their beliefs?

The next morning, after we had our first serving of Daime and settled into our seats, I noted that the fast-paced music that had been so jarring the day before felt soothing—uplifting, even. It was as though I had been on the outside looking in during the first day, but now I was plugged into the current of compassion.

My head and shoulders were swaying gently when I found myself joining in a hymn called "Porto Seguro," or "Safe Harbor."

My God
From the infinite
Hear my cry
My prayer of love

Because
You are my safe harbor
Only with you do I heal myself
And only with you I exist

You are light
That shines in all the universe
My father, I ask
For your strength

To sing
Is to leave darkness

Only with you I become safe
My Divine Lord

As the song ended, I basked in the radiant effect it had on me. The term *safe harbor* lingered in my mind, like a riddle, an invitation, an open door. As I looked around the yurt, contemplating the devout Daimistas, it seemed clear each had found a safe harbor in their faith in God, which was strengthened and reinforced through these rituals.

In my lifetime, church membership in the United States has taken a nosedive, from 71 percent in the 1980s to a record low of 47 percent in 2021, according to Gallup research. I was part of that trend, having grown up resolutely agnostic. My views on organized religion were shaped by the homophobia and hypocrisy I saw in the Catholic Church, the faith I was born into, and the violent expressions of Islam I witnessed as a journalist.

But suddenly, sitting in that light-filled yurt, I found myself seriously contemplating, perhaps for the first time, whether my irreligiosity had been a mistake. A 2019 study by the Pew Research Center found that in the United States, 36 percent of "actively religious" people describe themselves as "very happy," while 25 percent of people who described themselves as unaffiliated or inactively religious reported being very happy. Religious people also reported drinking and smoking less than nonpious folks; were more likely to be involved in other groups, like charities and clubs; and were more likely to vote.

How had I landed, seemingly by default and with little reflection, in the camp of nonbelievers? And what would it take to cross over, overriding the instincts, judgments, and assumptions about religion that had calcified within me over the years?

As I sat with those questions, a distant memory seized my attention. The final rite of passage of my short-lived tenure as a Catholic had been my confirmation, which took place when I was thirteen or fourteen, just entering puberty. I remembered virtually nothing about the ritual itself, other than the fact that I didn't see it as something I could avoid. But I vividly remembered two events that led up to it. My classmates and I spent the weekend before confirmation at a spiritual retreat held at a small lodge in the countryside, where there was a lot of prayer and obsessive warnings about a long list of things that were *pecados*—sins.

I was assigned to a room with a classmate named Carlos Andrés Díaz, a skinny boy with light brown hair. He'd never been friendly toward me—but I was enormously attracted to him. He said little to me during the two nights we shared a small room with two twin beds shrouded in red blankets. I lay awake at night, tormented by the intoxicating desire that can suddenly flood adolescent bodies. The profound loneliness of stifling what my body yearned to do, that night and many others, came roaring back to me as I remembered the scene.

Soon after we returned from the retreat, on the eve of confirmation, I found myself in a small office at school, where a priest was presiding over one final round of confession. He had white hair, pronounced bags under his eyes, and a dark brown robe.

"Have you had impure thoughts, my son?" he asked.

"Yes, Father," I replied, assuming I was in good company.

"Do you want to tell me more?" he continued.

After a pause, I replied, "No," and wondered if being evasive was also a bit sinful.

He nodded and told me how many Padre Nuestros and Ave Marias I needed to recite in order to be acquitted in time for confirmation the following day. I remember praying feverishly afterward, keeping a rigorous count to make sure my penance was absolved.

As I allowed that sequence of memories to unfurl gently, without resistance, I found myself feeling tremendous tenderness toward that version of myself, at once distant and somehow throbbingly alive. Had I found a path to regaining faith, to reimagining my relationship with God, to reconsidering Catholic symbols and teachings, embracing the valuable lessons they offer on love, redemption, and forgiveness?

Suddenly, I heard Jonathan say something about "Christ consciousness," and my attention shifted back to what was happening in the *salão* (hall). There's a danger in being overly doctrinaire about religious beliefs and practices, Jonathan said, particularly when they turn people off from the baseline notion that there is a higher power.

"Call it what you will—but *call it*," Jonathan exhorted. "Call it God, call it the creator, call it the numinous, call it the Divine Mother, call it the mystery."

In that moment, the last vestiges of judgment, skepticism, and unease I had walked in with the day before receded. Their absence created space for an incandescent sense of peace. And within it, I felt overflowing with love. Was this what it felt like to have faith in God, in a higher power, in Jonathan's so-called mystery?

Suddenly, it felt plausible—tempting, even—to expand the boundaries of my beliefs, to allow for the possibility that songs can be channeled from the realm of spirits; that some ailing souls get stuck somewhere between earth and the astral plane; that we can have a direct relationship with God, the numinous, the mystery—*call it what you will!*—and that cultivating it gives clarity to our thinking and purpose to our actions. On an impulse, I reached inside my tote bag and fished out a notebook. I felt an urge to write a couple of phrases that felt more streamed than inspired.

"We heal when we make peace with the thoughts that torment us," I wrote. "It takes practice to disarm them, to let them be, but quieter, gentler—until they are no more. And that is exactly what we are here on Earth to do. We're here to practice."

I read those words slowly over and over, each time finding a new layer of meaning. I loved them. I couldn't decide if they were merely the product of my imagination or the fruits of something otherworldly. But it didn't bother me. Call it a mystery.

11 THE NEW PSYCHEDELIC CHURCHES MINISTERING TO VETERANS

WHITNEY LASSETER WAS RAISED BY a devout Southern Baptist mother in Tennessee who dragged her to church on Sundays and to Bible school on Wednesdays. Her father was an atheist who found Zen in intense workouts. That spiritual dichotomy became a source of torment during Whitney's childhood, poisoning her views on organized religion for many years. "I hated going to church," Whitney told me. "I hated sitting still. And if what they were telling me was true, my dad was going to hell."

So she's the first to admit that the journey that led her to build a new congregation from scratch in early 2022, soon after moving to Austin, was circuitous, more an act of pragmatism and risk mitigation than divine inspiration.

By founding the All Tribes Medicine Assembly, which operates out of a five-bedroom house in a quiet residential neighborhood, Whitney joined scores of psychedelic practitioners who came to see registering as a church as a means of giving their practice a veneer of legal compliance, arguing that the case law established by the ayahuasca

churches should be understood to provide broad coverage to the sacramental use of psychedelics.

As their number and visibility grows, these churches have become
markers at the intersection of religious freedom protections and drug
policy, an unsettled area of the law that is being shaped by unusual
allies who include religious conservatives, veterans groups, and psychedelic enthusiasts. Taking comfort in the 2006 Supreme Court
ruling that opened the door for the legal use of ayahuasca in religious
rituals, scores of new psychedelic churches are hoping to radically
expand what is permissible under the law.

After the DEA was forced to establish a regulatory system enabling
Santo Daime and União do Vegetal members to import and consume their psychoactive sacrament, the agency established a system
for others wishing to apply for a religious exemption to federal drug
laws. However, lawyers who represent psychedelic practitioners say
the DEA has not approved a single petition filed since then. And
the process of applying puts practitioners in a bind: the application
must describe the intended use of drugs in ceremonial settings, but
petitioners are ordered to refrain from using controlled substances
while a case is pending.

Daniel Peterson, a lawyer in Washington, DC, who founded the
Association of Entheogenic Practitioners, which advises psychedelic churches, said the government's religious exemption process
effectively makes counternarcotics agents arbiters of what consti-
tutes sincere religious practice. "It's kind of a kangaroo court in that
they're saying that 'you should apply to us even though we have no
regulatory authority to do this and no institutional competence to
judge what is a religion,'" he said. "You're required to give all this
potential testimony against yourself and affirm that your intention
is to commit felonies."

The DEA did not respond to my requests for an interview about
psychedelic churches. But the agency has made clear it opposes a
more permissive regulatory landscape as part of a court battle the

federal government has been waging against an ayahuasca group in Orlando since 2020.

The group, called Soul Quest Ayahuasca Church of Mother Earth Inc., has been hosting weekend retreats out of a suburban home since 2016. It was among the first psychedelic communities in the United States to start operating openly under the cover of the 2006 ruling, spelling out the nature of its offerings online and inviting filmmakers to document its rituals. On its website, Soul Quest presents a forty-six-page holy text titled *Ayahuasca Manifesto: Ayahuasca and Its Planetary Mission*, which describes the dramatic expansion of ayahuasca as vital for the survival of the human race. "If I don't spread globally I will face extinction, similar to Humans," the manifesto proclaims. "For survival reasons, I must spread globally, while Humans must accept my sacred medicine to heal their afflicted soul and be able to achieve its divine destiny."

Soul Quest faced scrutiny from local and federal law enforcement officials following the April 2018 death of a twenty-two-year-old retreat participant who had a seizure following a kambo ceremony. But the death—which did not result in criminal charges—did little to dampen the group's crusading spirit. In 2020, Soul Quest sued the DEA, demanding a religious exemption, setting in motion the first of several contemporary legal battles over the permissible use of psychedelics in spiritual settings.

In a detailed letter denying Soul Quest's exemption request, the DEA argued that the group was a church on paper only. Its investigators concluded that retreat participants weren't expected to profess devotion to the ayahuasca manifesto and that the forms they filled out to become members of the church were meaningless. "Membership in Soul Quest appears to be purely a pro forma matter to obtain access to ayahuasca, rather than an expression of sincere religious devotion," the agency wrote. Notably, in its letter, the DEA cited the Oregon Santo Daime church as an example of a bona fide church, without alluding to the government's previous efforts to shut it down.

The DEA noted that Soul Quest promotes ayahuasca as a "natural remedy" for depression, anxiety, post-traumatic stress, and drug addiction. "This language from the website supports a conclusion that Soul Quest understands and advertises the use and distribution of ayahuasca to the public as fundamentally medicinal," the letter concluded. In the government's view, this was an alternative therapy masquerading as religion.

Despite the rejection and the lengthy investigation that preceded it, the federal government has so far refrained from filing criminal charges against Soul Quest's leaders. Nationally, federal and state officials have shown little appetite for prosecuting people who provide psychedelics in spiritual and therapeutic settings.

Anthony Coulson, a retired senior DEA agent, said psychedelics have become among the lowest enforcement priorities for the federal government for a couple of reasons. For starters, the agency is overwhelmed by the flood of opioids like fentanyl, powerfully addictive drugs that kill tens of thousands of people each year. And its experience going up against ayahuasca churches in the early 2000s made the DEA deeply reluctant to meddle in the thorny intersection of religious freedom law and drug policy. "They want to avoid it like the plague," Anthony told me.

That has emboldened many practitioners to begin operating in plain view—and has prompted a handful of others to go on a legal offensive. Since Soul Quest sued the DEA, two ayahuasca churches in Arizona have filed similar federal lawsuits seeking a religious exemption to drug laws.

Ian Benouis, an attorney in Texas who advises psychedelic churches, said it's a matter of time before one of these cases reaches the Supreme Court again. While many in the psychedelic space are socially and politically liberal, he and other lawyers in the field view the court's hardening conservative bent as a godsend. "This Supreme Court may accelerate the end of the war on drugs through these church cases," Ian said. "If this Supreme Court really believes in freedom of religion, freedom of worship, and all these freedoms we supposedly hold dear, it will give these churches the same protection."

∿∿ Much has changed since the Supreme Court last tackled this issue in 2006. The two churches that won the right to use ayahuasca as a sacrament in the 2000s were staunchly opposed to commodifying their sacrament. Their aversion to proselytizing kept the congregations small and largely inconspicuous. Their rituals were rooted in Christianity, and there was never any doubt that the emphasis was spiritual rather than therapeutic.

The new crop of psychedelic churches is emerging at a time of booming demand for therapeutic interventions with mind-altering drugs. Several were born out of an acknowledged desire to provide a veneer of legality to retreats and therapeutic practices that emerged in the underground. Some are strikingly flashy in their marketing and social media presence, hailing the transformational potential of psychedelics. Church websites list upcoming retreats along with their cost and offer the ability to pay with a credit card. Several of these new churches promote their work treating veterans, touting their services as an alternative to the overburdened and underperforming mental health care system.

Browsing the websites of these new psychedelic churches, I was captivated by the All Tribes Medicine Assembly, known as ATMA. In photos and videos, it came across as a wonderland for new age hippies. ATMA does not have a manifesto or allegiance to any religious lineage or text. Its main worship space—once a living room—features crosses, Buddha statues, and Indigenous art. "We Are a Sanctuary of Souls Experiencing Heaven on Earth," the church's website proclaims.

Seconds after I texted the number listed on the website, Whitney and I were on the phone. I expected, given the legally dubious nature of her work, that she would be guarded speaking to a reporter. But from the beginning, she was warm, funny, and candid to a fault. She would later tell me that she has come to trust that the right people and opportunities drift into her orbit because she keeps her vibrations high.

So when I reached out, her intuition signaled that it was a good omen, that our lives had been meant to intersect, that our relationship would serve a higher purpose. My own intuition suggested that Whitney meant well but may have been in over her head. The church's finances were a nightmare, she said; figuring out its mission and purpose remained very much a work in progress.

Whitney suggested I come visit during the Halloween weekend extravaganza: she was planning to hire a magician, have guests paint pumpkins while smoking pot, and the grand finale would be a ceremony with a psychoactive cactus called huachuma. I was fascinated. What kind of person decides to open a psychedelic church?

〰〰 Whitney was born in 1979 in Murfreesboro, a small city on the outskirts of Nashville. Raised by doting parents who "loved me and spoiled me," Whitney said she felt like a misfit from an early age. She began smoking marijuana in high school, then developed a liking for Xanax, which she stole from a friend's mother. Soon, Whitney got her hands on LSD, a drug that augmented her rebellious streak.

"Doing these massive amounts of acid, I began having some revelations," she told me. "Even at that young age, I concluded that it doesn't matter what anybody thinks."

During her freshman year of high school, Whitney checked into rehab for the first of several attempts to get sober. But after getting out, she picked up a cocaine habit and became pregnant at sixteen. When her son was born, Whitney began doing crack, often purchased with money she stole from her parents. Soon after graduating from high school, she got pregnant again, at twenty. One day, desperate to get high, she bought an ounce of crack. Barefoot, disheveled, and with the drug in hand, she walked into a gas station to pick up lighters and five Brillo pads, which are used to make pipes. When she turned around, Whitney locked eyes with a police officer. She was arrested and faced felony charges. Realizing how much harm crack was doing to her body, Whitney shifted to a new drug: ecstasy.

Her low point with drug use came when Whitney was in her early twenties, living in Florida. She overdosed on GHB, also known as the date rape drug, in a parking lot of a bar. A nurse spotted her as she lay passed out and rendered aid while paramedics arrived. "My left lung collapsed when they were trying to resuscitate me," Whitney told me. "I flatlined for thirty seconds."

Regaining consciousness following what she described as a close brush with death, Whitney experienced something of a rebirth. "I'd had this deep hatred for myself, for everyone, and that was gone," she said. "I started having this deep sense of love and connection for others and seeing that there was a higher purpose."

After that, Whitney turned her life around. She began working out compulsively and started making a decent living stripping at nightclubs and working as a personal trainer at a retirement home. During her midthirties, she spent a couple of years traversing the country in an RV with a pizza oven repairman she fell madly in love with. Their breakup plunged Whitney into a period of heartache that felt unshakable. She turned to a mysterious drug derived from toad venom that had become popular among spiritual seekers. People often describe their first hit of the drug, which is known as Bufo and 5-MeO-DMT, as a dazzling burst of divinity. Bufo smokers emerge from the short-lasting trips making hyperbolic claims about seeing God, experiencing an exorcism, or realizing that heaven is accessible to mortals. So it was for Whitney.

"It was, like, everything," Whitney said. "I understood who I was. I understood why I had gone through all I had gone through." It made her believe that all the stumbles had been lessons she needed to learn in this lifetime, trials by fire to prepare her for a life of service.

Soon after discovering Bufo, Whitney traveled to Mexico, where she briefly lived with a family that taught her how to administer the powerful drug. She then set up an underground Bufo practice in Jupiter, Florida, treating people for depression and anxiety. Early in the pandemic, itching for a change of scenery, she bought an RV using a $50,000 loan from a federal government economic incentive program and drove to Austin. In the Texas capital, she befriended fellow psychedelic enthusiasts, and her Bufo practice, operating out of the mobile home, took off. As her profile grew, a friend advised her to file paperwork to register as a church, arguing that it would make risky work a bit safer. Whitney said it suddenly clicked: in her recent personal Bufo ceremonies, she had been seeing visions of people coming together, of leading an effort to stitch back the fabric of community in a world full of lonely people. "We need to have community," she recalled thinking at the time. "We need to be celebrating being alive. We need to erupt in ecstatic praise."

Whitney had virtually no savings and plenty of credit card debt, but she scraped together enough money to cover the attorney and filing fees to register ATMA as a church in the state. The $10,000 monthly rent plus maintenance costs she had taken on felt like a stretch. But the means kept materializing at the right time. Two new Austin friends who were inspired by Whitney's vision donated $5,000 each. Scores of locals signed up for the $55 monthly membership program, becoming "ATMA Angels." That provides access to Soul Tribe Sunday, the weekly service, along with discounted admission to special events and parties. Members get to use Whitney's backyard ice plunge container, inflatable hot tub, and barrel sauna, core components of her "human optimization" routine. But ATMA's main draw is that it offers people a chance to take a broad range of psychedelics in a group setting. When I asked Whitney how much she worried about the legal peril inherent in her work, her response made me think she would almost welcome a showdown. "I am willing to take the risk because I know I'm doing good work," she said. "I've seen lives change. I'm willing to be a martyr for the cause."

Whitney envisions a not-too-distant future in which there is broad agreement that certain drugs that have been prohibited for decades are tools of spiritual enlightenment and emotional healing. But Whitney worries, of course, about what may unfold if the cops show up one day. Which is why it seemed like a stroke of luck when two grizzled, traumatized marines found their way to her late in the summer of 2022. The men had both soured on the bureaucracy and treatment plans at the Department of Veterans Affairs. Both had come close to killing themselves. They were barely getting through the day when one got Whitney's number from a trusted contact and called to ask about upcoming retreats. Instantly, Whitney saw an opportunity. She could shift the focus of her church to treat veterans who are hurting—and the presence of the veterans, in turn, would help her church. If she were to face drug charges, she told me, there would be no shortage of veterans willing to testify in her defense.

〰〰 The first veterans to come to ATMA for treatment were Gary Hess and Joe Rovnak, longtime friends who met as marines during the war in Iraq. Both struggled with post-traumatic stress disorder after leaving the military and in recent years had found a slight reprieve in cannabis, they said. But years of therapy, antidepressants, and heavy drinking had done little to squash the demons of combat, which had turned swashbuckling warriors into chronically sleep-deprived, foggy-headed zombies. By the time Gary got Whitney on the phone, he was desperate to try something radically new. His marriage was in trouble. He woke up and went to bed every day stewing with rage. The fact that Whitney had no mainstream health care credentials actually felt like an asset. "You have two guys who have already sat with every doctor possible," Gary told me. "And their answers are not working. Honestly, we were out of options."

Gary joined the Marine Corps in February 1998, and early in his military career, America went to war. In 2005, he was deployed to a small outpost in western Iraq near the Syrian border, where the members of his unit got into more than 300 firefights over the course of 180 days. The worst day of that deployment was March 21, 2005, when a suicide bomber rammed into Gary's vehicle. A slab of shrapnel decapitated Gary's gunner and wounded the three other marines in the truck. Two would later kill themselves. "I've lost more marines to suicide than I did in combat," Gary told me. "And that's not a small number."

Of all the carnage he witnessed, the images that would haunt him for years came from an attack on December 26, 2006, during his second Iraq deployment. Gary was leading a small team operating out of a fortified house when the building was rammed by a dump truck laden with explosives. Gary remembers meeting the driver's eyes and hearing a thundering blast before losing consciousness. When Gary's eyes blinked open, he was stunned and relieved to be alive. Then he walked up to the rooftop. Josh, a young marine who had become a workout partner and close confidant, lay sprawled on his back. Next to him was brain matter. It reminded Gary of spilled macaroni.

"I picked up every piece of him to make sure he got home," Gary told me. He didn't know it then, but for years to come, the sight of macaroni would bring him back to that moment, to collecting the mangled corpse, inducing dread so severe Gary avoided anywhere macaroni might be served. "How do you tell people you're afraid of macaroni?" he told me. "That was the beginning of the end for me."

After leaving the military in 2008, Gary sought treatment at the VA. Doctors prescribed Adderall to get his mind to focus in the morning, antidepressants to taper compulsive thoughts, and Ambien to get him to sleep. The medications killed his libido and made Gary feel numb. And they didn't help. "They're treating the physical manifestations; they're not treating the root of the problem," he said. The fears and flashbacks worsened over the years, making Gary feel trapped. "There were times where I would get in the shower in the morning and sing 'Jesus Loves Me' out loud just to be louder than the voices in my head," he said. As his mood worsened, Gary retreated from his family and work. "Pretty soon, I was in a small house, just me and my dog," he said. He concluded, after much agonizing thought, that a self-inflicted gunshot was the only way out. "It wasn't out of impulse; it was out of exhaustion."

〰〰 Joe told me he joined the Marine Corps after a traumatic child-hood. His mother died on his ninth birthday. His father, a former marine, had been physically and emotionally abusive to his children, Joe said. When his sister got cancer at thirteen, Joe, who was sixteen, became her primary caretaker. After graduating from high school, he desperately wanted to go to art school, but had no way of paying for it. So he followed in his father's footsteps and enlisted. Joe said he volunteered eagerly and often for combat tours, compelled by a duty to put himself in situations "where I had to participate in and witness the worst humanity has to offer." Some memories stand out. There was the remains of a man who was run over by a tank, his brain splattered on asphalt. He remembers tending to elderly wounded Iraqi prisoners during the first Gulf War, including one whose scrotum had been blown off. But the most searing, by far, was the brief conversation he had with a marine he loved, Lance Corporal Lawrence Philippon, in early May 2005 during a deployment in Iraq.

"First Sergeant, you got a minute?" Joe remembers the twenty-two-year-old marine asking.

"I always got a minute for you," Joe replied. He lit a cigarette and sat next to him on a bench.

Larry confided that he had "a bad feeling" about a dangerous mission the following morning. "I don't know how to lead these guys," the young marine said. Joe didn't think twice. "Larry, tomorrow you're going to go and you're going to do what you need to do," Joe remembers having said. "You're going to kick in that door and those men are going to follow you, and you're going to execute your mission well. You're not even going to have to think about it. It's just going to happen."

The next day, Larry kicked in the door of a house that was a suspected insurgent hideout and got shot in the face. Joe had lost plenty of marines. But this loss was gutting.

"On that bench, there was a father in me that wanted to say, 'Larry, don't take any unnecessary chances. Keep your men safe,'" Joe told me. "And he didn't; the marine spoke up. And that was a moral injury that I carried with me for a long time. Every day, I thought about that conversation with that kid who trusted me."

Joe left the Marine Corps in 2007, having concluded, reluctantly, that he could no longer be an effective warrior. He joined the Defense Intelligence Agency, the Pentagon's intelligence division, as a civilian, seeing it as an opportunity to continue serving his country away from the battlefields. "When Larry died, I knew I was compromised," Joe explained. "Sometimes you have to be willing to lose a few guys to prevent future battles, and I didn't have that in me anymore."

Joe said he went to therapy after leaving the military and was treated for post-traumatic stress. But over the years, the losses and horrors he had seen swirled through his mind with growing intensity. He came to think of his invisible wounds as the stench of a skunk. "You get sprayed by a skunk, and those clothes, you can wash them a thousand times, and that stench doesn't leave you," he said. "That's kind of how I felt for a long time as I carried that stench on me that nobody else could smell or see."

He was a competent and committed intelligence officer, but over the years, as the job gave him a broader vantage point of geopolitics and military operations, he became increasingly conflicted and cynical. "They're sending innocent people in harm's way, and they're sending people to do things that are hurting them for the rest of their lives," Joe said. "I began to feel more and more like a pawn in a sick man's game."

Having participated in the invasion of Panama in 1989, the Gulf War in Kuwait, and the Iraq War, Joe was no stranger to fraught, high-stakes missions. But the chaotic, bloody exit of American forces from Afghanistan in the summer of 2021 broke him, Joe said. His face broke out with psoriasis. He began throwing up every morning and experienced chronic diarrhea. Driving to work became impossible as his hands trembled. Joe went on medical disability for a while, but the symptoms only worsened. "I was trying to figure out how to kill myself and make it look like an accident so that everybody would get their insurance cut," Joe told me.

Gary, a longtime friend, recognized that Joe was spiraling and flew to check in on him. Having found relief in cannabis, Gary offered some to Joe, who initially refused, citing his lifelong aversion to drugs and the fact that smoking pot was a violation of his security clearance. But one day he relented, smoked some weed, and for the first time in years, slept soundly through the night. Before leaving, Gary left Joe a chocolate bar infused with psilocybin and planted the seeds of an idea: Was it time to consider a psychedelic retreat?

Joe ate the bar one morning on an empty stomach. Within minutes, he sprang up with a sudden desire to tend to his neglected yard. Looking up, he was moved by the beauty of the cloudless sky, and marveled at the ability, at long last, to feel something other than anguish. He called Gary to tell him he was ready to try something stronger. *I'll at least die trying, if it kills me*, Joe recalled thinking.

〰️ The first thing Whitney did when Joe and Gary walked into her house in August 2022 was wash their feet. It was a gesture of devotion and humility toward the ailing warriors who had found their way to her, and the start of their retreat. The protocol she uses to treat veterans unfolds over the course of three days and includes three main ceremonies held in a room that has a giant Golden Buddha statue, crucifixes, and a large mandala with images of snakes that hangs over a fireplace.

The first major ceremony is intended to detoxify. After drinking a lot of water, participants are treated with kambo, the medicine derived from the poisonous secretions of a frog, which induces a state of bloat and malaise that is alleviated by intense vomiting. On the second day, veterans are given a large dose of magic mushrooms mixed into a hot cacao drink. After drinking the brew, they lie on mats arranged in a U-shape on the floor wearing eyeshades and noise-canceling earphones. As the effects kick in, participants often cry, spasm, and flail their arms as though they are navigating a different reality. Whitney and her assistant facilitator, Dani Amelio, move around the room gingerly, often taking a knee next to a participant who appears to be struggling. Sometimes they hold their hands; sometimes they caress their necks; sometimes they provide a long, tender embrace. During the final ceremony, participants smoke Bufo, the toad venom that contains a potent form of DMT.

Taking a major dose of psilocybin for the first time, Gary said he was terrified as his thoughts drifted to the day of the dump truck bombing. But having somehow surrendered to the fear, something unimaginable happened. He saw himself, in crisp detail, sitting next to the suicide bomber who had killed his friend and mangled his mind. Inside the cabin of that truck, loaded with explosives, the two men had a conversation and acknowledged each other as fighters in a war, merely doing what more powerful people had tasked them to do. "I had to respect him. I had to understand him and understand everything he did," Gary told me. "We both presented ourselves on the battlefield, as warriors." Gary said he then sat with a fifteen-year-old girl his unit shot one day after mistakenly identifying the vehicle she was in as a threat. He saw himself standing on the roof with Larry minutes before the bomb detonated, and offering to trade places with the young marine—a proposal the young man turned down. Gary said he felt as though a higher force were guiding him to view key moments of the war from the perspective of others in a manner that mysteriously deflated their traumatic imprint. "It gives you a new understanding that absolutely releases the chains," Gary said. "Emotions are still felt, but it doesn't carry the weight that it did in the past."

Whitney had told Gary that the key to healing was reconnecting with the feeling of love. The idea had struck him as Pollyannaish. Now it made sense. His capacity to love had grown so boundless it extended even to the suicide bomber. "I had so much love and appreciation for that guy," Gary said, chuckling. "It doesn't sound reasonable."

Reasonable or not, soon the sight of macaroni didn't make him recoil.

Sitting just a few feet from Gary during the mushroom ceremony, Joe was having a similarly perspective-bending trip. He saw himself as the center of attention at a fancy gathering attended by relatives and magnificent beings, including an Egyptian priestess, who spanned many eras of human history. His mother, long deceased, was present and looking at Joe with love. There were people in pastel polyester suits. Maybe this was a wedding, Joe remembered thinking. Then a shaman "with an ancient face and tribal markings and bones woven into his hair" appeared on his left. On his right was a young, imposing warrior with similar tribal markings. As the men led Joe to the center of the hall, dread rippled through his body as he grasped the nature of the proceedings. "This was my trial," Joe said. "It was judgment day." Joe said he felt tremendously exposed, feeling that he was surrounded by a massive crowd that could see everything he had ever said, done, and thought. When the crowd grew silent, Joe steeled himself for a reckoning. But the elders in the room began clapping. "You have such a pure heart, Joe," he remembers one elder proclaiming. "Not only was I acquitted, I was applauded."

〰〰 Joe and Gary left ATMA feeling dazzled. It felt as though they had somehow been pulled out of a sinkhole of hopelessness. The two veterans, who had long held a dim view of drug users, suddenly became evangelists for the healing power of psychedelics and ambassadors of Whitney's start-up church. Having both lost several comrades to suicide, they began making a list of fellow veterans who appeared to be on the brink. Robert, the former soldier from Illinois who came close to killing himself, was a priority case. I had initially planned to visit Whitney's church to attend a two-day Halloween event that on paper sounded like a spectacle. But four days before my flight, Whitney suggested I travel sooner to observe a last-minute veterans' retreat. She had squeezed it into her schedule after hearing

the story about Robert, the gun in his mouth, and the brief hospitalization that left him even more destabilized.

Robert grew up in Barrington, Illinois, a wealthy suburb of Chicago,
and was raised by a divorced mother who worked three jobs to provide
for the family. When he graduated from high school, Robert wanted
to go to culinary school and turn his passion for cooking into a career.
But in 2005, fresh out of high school and with America awash in patri-
otic fervor in the early years of its wars in Afghanistan and Iraq, Robert
walked into an army recruitment office and filled out an application.
"I had red, white, and blue in my eyes," he told me.

He deployed to Iraq in the summer of 2006, assigned to a violent
district southwest of Baghdad, where his unit was pushed into insurgent strongholds that had not seen American combat troops. They
were almost giddy with excitement during their first firefight, Robert
said. But within days, soldiers in his unit began succumbing to small
arms fire and roadside bombs, and "it became a different game."

On January 7, 2007, as Robert's platoon was trying to draw out
insurgent snipers who had killed a couple of American troops in the
area, a bullet from a Russian-made Dragunov rifle pierced Robert's
arm. After recovering, he was given the option of going home, but he
chose not to cut the eighteen-month deployment short. "I went back
to the field," he said, "and we just had casualty after casualty."

One attack haunts him. A vehicle transporting four US Military
Police troops who were delivering supplies at his small base was
hit by a roadside bomb. The truck had cans of .50-caliber rounds,
which went off for minutes, an agonizing series of pops that made it
impossible to approach the vehicle to retrieve the charred soldiers.
"You could just smell these four guys," he said. "And you couldn't
do anything."

When they returned home to Fort Drum in New York, Robert and
his fellow soldiers underwent routine psychiatric evaluations. Everyone knew not to show signs of trauma, he said, because it was widely
assumed that doing so was a kiss of death for infantry careers. "If you
answer anything wrong, you're a pussy," he said.

But they were scarred by the bloodshed they had witnessed. And they were mourning the friends they'd lost. "I drank a ton," he told me. "Everyone in the barracks was talking about what had happened, drowning themselves in bottles."

Robert realized Iraq had fundamentally changed him when his sister pulled him aside one day at a bar and told him how worried she was by his sullen demeanor. "I don't know what you've done with my brother, but I want him back," he remembered her saying.

After leaving the army in 2010, Robert continued to soothe his nerves by drinking heavily. He went to the VA for help and tried everything: therapy, treatment for traumatic brain injury, antidepressants, and antianxiety drugs. But he disliked the way the drugs made him feel.

"Every single therapist I talked to was the exact same thing, like they were reading from a fucking script," he said. "It was just medication after medication."

Robert got married, had three kids, and made a living as a diver working in underwater construction projects. Still struggling to ease into civilian life, he and a few veteran friends drew up plans for a nonprofit organization to organize retreats and events designed to foster the sense of community and purpose that members of the military often lose when they leave the service.

Plans for the group were starting to take shape when the chaotic American withdrawal from Afghanistan in August 2021 upended its mission. Overnight, Robert joined the patchwork of veteran organizations and informal networks that embarked on a mad scramble to evacuate Afghan allies as the Taliban took control of the country. He sent money to people in Kabul and Mazar-i-Sharif, a city in the north, intending to help Afghans with connections to the American government get to safe houses and ultimately board a flight to go abroad. It was impossible to discern between people who had the ability to shepherd vulnerable Afghans to safety and unscrupulous actors who saw an opportunity to fleece well-meaning Americans at the twilight of the corruption-plagued war. "Organizations were just pouring in money without due diligence," Robert said. "Everyone's wheels had to be greased."

During those frantic days, when thousands of Afghans were looking for a way out, Robert's cell phone number began circulating widely. Desperate pleas poured in. Afghans begged for help in scores of messages, often accompanied by photos and videos that were said to depict torture scars. His group had assumed responsibility for thirty-five families that were in hiding, awaiting a chance to go abroad. But there were thousands desperate to flee. "If you heard those voices," he told me, choking up. "I'd wake up and there'd be fifty-three messages and phone calls and voice messages."

As the dust settled over the evacuation, squabbles emerged over where much of the money spent trying to evacuate people had gone. It soon became apparent that much of it had been stolen. Some of the Afghans Robert had done business with started demanding more money, but it was impossible to ascertain who was grifting and who was presenting a rightful claim.

Robert's downward spiral accelerated. Shortly before the Afghanistan drawdown upended his life, Robert told me he had begun having "these wicked thoughts in my head that I wasn't going to be around next year."

After the frantic final days of the war, the thoughts became more pernicious. The question of why he would kill himself, curiously, was an afterthought, Robert said. "I became obsessed with how I was going to end my life." He considered how the carotid artery needed to be punctured to guarantee he would bleed out. He researched how fast a car would need to be going to ensure a fatal crash barreling into a tree. He contemplated shooting his femoral artery at a shooting range. He wondered if taking multiple vaccines in one day would induce a heart attack. "Even knowing what it would do to my three beautiful children, knowing the consequences, I still felt like it was a better option," he said.

After his attempt at the park failed, his family wrestled with what kind of help Robert needed. He had spent a short time at a hospital on suicide watch, but the experience did more to traumatize than stabilize him. "You have no phone, you can't talk to anybody, you can't have your personal items," he said. "There's one TV for forty-five people that are walking around drugged up on medication. It's not a place for healing."

Robert and his family considered inpatient programs and trying antidepressants again, neither of which were appealing. Then his brother-in-law, a fellow veteran, mentioned a woman in Austin whom veteran friends had been raving about. Given how many crazy things had happened over the past year, somehow booking a last-minute slot for one of Whitney's retreats seemed like a good idea. He wired the $2,888 fee.

∿∿ Before putting on his eyeshades for the psilocybin session, Robert jotted down a few final thoughts in his journal. Whitney had guided him through an exercise to set a clear intention, to define what they wanted to attain. He had come up with three words: *joy*, *freedom*, and *stability*. As he was about to gulp down the brew, Robert penned the following question on a blank page: "Did I find it?"

A few hours into the session, lying on his back, Robert flailed his hands in the air as though he were touching something. At one point, I noticed him crying. Then there was a broad smile. Whitney and Dani took turns tending to him, resting their palms on his chest, holding his hand. I was struck by the certainty they bring to their work, but also by the love and devotion they show people who are hurting.

Later, he would describe feeling that his hands were "dredging really angry energy" from his body and pushing it out and "Whitney was just there to take it."

Suddenly, upon hearing the first note of a harp song, he felt a spasm, like something within him had unclenched. "I was in pure nirvana," he said. "Pure happiness."

With his blindfold still on, Robert reached for his journal and, next to the question he had left himself a couple of hours earlier, scribbled in huge letters: *YES*.

When we spoke the next day, Robert told me his journeys had not dredged up traumatic memories or taken him to dreamlike scenes like Gary and Joe described. He told me he had experienced his healing on what he called "the other side, another realm," for which there is no vocabulary. But something had become clear, he said. He felt enthralled to be alive and relieved he hadn't shot himself in that parking lot, "leaving my wife without a husband, my kids without a father, my mother without a son."

Spending hours listening to these stories dredged up some of my old demons related to war. Having never experienced armed conflict as a combatant, I had never carefully considered the extent to which war had scarred me. But that changed once I began drinking ayahuasca.

12 REMINISCING ON MY WARS

WITH OUR HIGH SCHOOL GRADUATION a few months away in 1999, the boys in my senior class at Colegio Nueva Granada in Bogotá gathered in a cold gymnasium for a perfunctory physical exam conducted by the army to assess our fitness for a year of compulsory military service.

Standing side by side a couple of feet apart, we faced a gruff officer in fatigues who barked out orders. As a couple of male doctors put on surgical gloves, we were instructed to strip down to our underwear. Once our clothes were piled up on the floor, the doctors made their way down the line, moving from left to right. They scanned each body for obvious abnormalities, gently felt the lymph nodes in our necks, and pressed the cold diaphragm of a stethoscope against our chests to listen to our agitated hearts. Then came the final, demeaning step. Each of us had to drop our briefs so a physician could feel our testicles, then turn our heads left and cough, ostensibly to screen us for hernias, before advancing to the next student.

The symbolism of that gesture was unmistakable: they had us by the balls. At a particularly bloody juncture of Colombia's decades-long armed conflict, each of us could conceivably be thrown into the front lines of a sprawling war that included guerrilla fighters, powerful drug cartels, and right-wing paramilitary groups that often worked in concert with the state. The country's violence had shaped and circumscribed our lives from birth. Bloodshed and threats had most profoundly ravaged rural communities, displacing millions, but by the time we approached adulthood, the conflict had permeated all the major cities. We could not ignore it or escape it.

Several students in my school had a parent who had been abducted for ransom, and kidnapping insurance had become a necessary expense for moneyed families. Some of my wealthy classmates had left Colombia abruptly during our final years of school as families with the means had sought refuge abroad. At the mountainside campus of my private school, classes were occasionally interrupted by loud blasts. The sound sent us racing to the nearest lookout point, where we would scan a sea of redbrick buildings looking for a plume of dark gray smoke.

Despite the barbarity unfolding around us, my classmates and I, having attended Colombia's premier American school, recognized that we had grown up with enormous privilege. Many of us lived in heavily secured homes, on streets where neighbors invested in private armed guards and sophisticated alarm systems. Several of us were applying for college abroad, taking advantage of our bilingual education. And yet here were these dour military men to remind us that in a wartime nation with military conscription for men, under the law, there were limits to our entitlement.

During a presentation held at our school soon after the physical exam, an officer with a pronounced belly stood behind a podium to issue a stern warning. Surely, he said, many of us assumed that we could buy our way out of this duty. Surely we had heard that there had long been an all-but-institutionalized system of bribes that ensured that Colombia's poor would continue bearing the brunt of the fighting, their lost lives and limbs further dragging down some of the nation's neediest families. But the army had cracked down, he claimed, and this year, there would be absolutely no room for kickbacks, no way to skirt our lawful duty to wear the uniform if we were deemed physically fit and able to bolster the ranks of the state.

〜〜 I hadn't had reason to reminisce on those dreadful days for decades when they roared back during an ayahuasca ceremony in early 2020 at a new retreat center in the mountains outside Rio de Janeiro. The memory surfaced with the intensity of a boisterous, unwelcome guest who shows up at your door unannounced and refuses to leave until he has said his piece. This was not the first time I had been plunged into a distressing sequence of memories after downing a big serving of ayahuasca, and by now, I knew better than to resist.

The first inkling that the theme of war would be taking center stage came in a couple of words in Spanish that began cycling through my mind on a loop. *Patria ensangrentada.* Blood-drenched homeland. The turn of phrase is one I likely had encountered before, perhaps in a headline or a quote, but there was nothing specific I associated it with. At this point in my life, approaching forty, Colombia's conflict seemed to occupy little room in my mind. I had left the country more than two decades earlier. The main guerrilla group, the FARC, had signed a peace deal with the government. I'd moved on, covered other wars, and had little reason to dwell on that bygone era. It had been awful, certainly, but was of ever-diminishing consequence to me. So why was I being invited—commanded, perhaps—to reopen this dusty drawer and examine its contents?

Secuestro. That was far and away my biggest fear growing up. From infancy, I had become acutely aware that kidnappings were fair game. Politicians were abducted while campaigning. Soldiers taken hostage on the battlefield were kept in cages, often with chains on their necks for good measure. Haunting footage of their inhumane treatment was broadcast on the news.

Wealthy Colombians were seized in their fincas, or country homes, by guerrilla groups that were at war with elites they regarded, not without reason, as oligarchs who had kept a tight grip on land, wealth, and opportunity for generations. By the time I was a teenager, kidnapping had become so pervasive there was a popular radio show called *Voces del Secuestro—Voices of Kidnapping—*during which relatives of people who had been abducted called the station and were given a few minutes to speak to their missing loved ones. The messages, tender, searing, at once desperate and hopeful, were beamed to an audience of hundreds of thousands. The hope—often realized—was that among them would be the intended recipient, somewhere in a jungle hideout, holding up a scratchy radio, and finding in it connection to a life suddenly usurped.

On road trips, we were wary of stumbling into a *pesca milagrosa*—a biblical term for a miraculous catch of fish, which, in war parlance, referred to mass kidnappings carried out in remote roads. During those operations, captors blocked a long strip of road at gunpoint, stopped vehicles, and made a quick assessment of the wealth and status of the terrified occupants as they decided which ones to take deep into the jungle for an extended *secuestro.*

The threat of kidnapping cast a shadow over a plot of land my parents had bought when I was thirteen or so in a mountainous area about an hour away from Bogotá. When we acquired it, the area, so close to the capital, felt well within the urban buffer zone believed to be beyond the reach of the guerrillas. My father bought four off-road motorcycles, built an outdoor brick oven to make fresh bread, and made tentative plans to build a comfortable house near the highest point of the property, which has a sweeping view of the nearby lake and surrounding valley. But just a few months after we acquired it, a close call filled us with dread and cast a dark shadow over a place we had hoped would be a refuge.

A friend and I had gone there for a weekend to camp. At night, we marveled at the starlit sky, cooked sausages on a small grill, and wondered aloud about a helicopter that swooped in and out of the valley below around midnight. We woke up soon after dawn the next morning. The surrounding field of unkempt grass sparkled with dew.

Shivering, I set out to reignite our campfire. Struggling to set a fresh log ablaze, I heard a low rumble from a truck lumbering up a dirt road that runs alongside one of the borders of the property. The flatbed was packed with men in camouflage uniforms. It came to a stop, and the men, a dozen or so, jumped out, crossed into our property, and began running toward us.

"*¡Guerrilla!*" I cried out.

A jolt of adrenaline made me leap onto one of the dirt bikes, which we had left by the tent. My friend followed suit. I kick-started the engine with my bare foot and barreled downhill as the heavily armed men in uniform gave chase, screaming words I couldn't decipher. There were two sections of the property cordoned off with a barbed wire fence, and when I hit the first obstacle, I thought little about blasting a hole through it with the bike. That's when I heard the first pop. It took a few seconds to register that we were under fire. It didn't occur to me to stop and surrender. I was in fight-or-flight mode, clearly outgunned and determined to avoid being kidnapped.

Within three minutes, we made it down to the main entrance of the property, where a family of caretakers had a modest home. I ran into their house screaming, asking for a place to hide. My memory is foggy about the sequence of events that followed. But soon, it became clear that the gunmen were soldiers, not guerrilla fighters. At the time, the army and the members of the two main guerrilla groups, the FARC and the ELN, wore similar uniforms.

There hadn't been any reason the army would enter our property unannounced, hence my default assumption that the operation was a *secuestro*. But the whole thing had been a mistaken counternarcotics operation, they explained. The helicopter we had heard the night before, we were later told, was suspected of picking up bricks of cocaine that were then flown to Panama. A surveillance team had spotted our campsite the day before and assumed it was a drug-smuggling staging ground.

The soldiers, realizing how close they had come to killing two innocent teenagers, left the property quickly.

〰〰 My memory of the days that followed is spotty. I remember clearly that my mother asked me not to tell my sisters what had happened, "*para no asustarlas*," so as to not scare them. She wrote a letter to the First Lady at the time, Ana Milena Muñoz de Gaviria, whom she had met socially, lodging a formal complaint. I returned to the finca the following week with Mónica Rodriguez, a friend of the family who was a prominent television journalist. She had me reenact the escape for the cameras, and if memory serves, her report noted that two army commanders had been suspended. I don't recall if we ever got a more formal response or apology from the government. Colombia back then was such a lawless, trigger-happy place; crimes and mistakes, big and small, went unpunished. *Patria ensangrentada.*

A few years earlier, we had had another close call, which I found my mind drifting to next. I was returning home from a haircut with my mother, and after ringing the doorbell, we spotted unusual activity in the foyer. I remember seeing our nanny, Catalina, who kept her thinning gray hair in a bun, sitting on the floor, face down, while three strange men paced around. Soon after the door opened, my dad, speaking gravely, informed us a home invasion was underway and we were instructed to kneel on the floor, do whatever the men asked, and refrain from looking at their faces. Time ticked by at an agonizing pace as the gunmen packed our television sets and the Betamax we used to watch American movies into the trunk of a car parked outside. They emptied my mother's jewelry into a bag. My father pointed to a hiding place where he kept cash in dollars and in pesos. My father led the gunmen to his closet, where he kept two firearms and boxes of ammunition, which they gladly took.

One of the gunmen kept asking for our safe. We didn't have one. My father tried to appease him by pointing to valuable art. The man demanded the safe. If we held back, he said, they would take my younger sister, Alicia, who was one or two at the time. Shortly before they left, he pointed to a framed photo of me at Disney World, smiling and wearing a baseball cap with Mickey Mouse ears. He said his children would also like to go to Disney World, which at the time seemed like an absurd thing to say. But as I revisited that offhand remark, it occurred to me that it spoke to the entrenched inequality, and the resentment it generated, which had been at the heart of Colombia's war.

When the men left, Catalina ran to the kitchen and pulled a pot of blackened french fries that had been burning on the stove during the entire ordeal. I remembered how it smelled in the kitchen and wondered if we ended up eating anything that night. The gunmen had ordered us not to call the police, but a few minutes after they sped off with our belongings, one of my parents called. When the cops arrived, I remember one of them saying these sorts of crimes were nearly impossible to solve. We had been lucky, they said. No one had been harmed. *Patria ensangrentada.*

I don't recall either of these events looming large in my mind in my final weeks of high school, while I worried about being drafted into the army. I conferred with classmates, and my mother consulted with other parents as we explored options. I remember reading somewhere that being openly gay would be a disqualifying strike, a lawful way out. But at the time, I had a girlfriend, and coming out was scarier than going to war.

Soon, we got word that there was a woman who had been visiting the homes of classmates, offering to broker a waiver from the army in exchange for cash. I don't recall how we determined this woman was trustworthy, but one afternoon, she was sitting in our living room sipping tea. She spoke fast and had a dry sense of humor. She told us it used to be a lot cheaper to get out of service but that many hands had to be greased now. Her price was nonnegotiable: buying my way out of serving in the military would cost eight million pesos—about $8,600, adjusted for inflation. In cash.

If I saw the money exchange hands, I don't recall. But I know she was paid. By the time I collected my diploma, my military service requirement was listed as fulfilled, and I was issued an official government card with my photo attesting to that. Of my graduating class of about one hundred, I can think of only three who enlisted. I recently asked one, Carlos Andrés Díaz—the same classmate I had shared a room with during the high school confirmation retreat—why he chose to serve. He was well aware most of us were planning to pay bribes. But at the time, he explained, he was trying desperately to suppress his attraction to men and saw in military service a means to overcome unwanted desires.

"I wouldn't allow myself to be gay," Carlos, who would later come out of the closet, told me. "I wanted to prove that I was a man."

Reflecting on that bribe and the shame associated with it—which had been deeply repressed in my memory bank—triggered an unbearable bout of nausea that left me curled in the fetal position in the ceremony room. I knew that inequality and corruption had long been Colombia's foundational problems, the fuel of its violence. But until then, I had never considered my own role in the country's war. Was I a victim, one of the millions of Colombians who grew up in a state of terror? After all, the army nearly shot me when I was a teenager. Or was I among the war's many culprits? And did grappling with these questions more than two decades later even matter?

Patria ensangrentada. Patria ensangrentada. Patria ensangrentada. With these words swirling through my mind, I leaped to my feet and vomited. Afterward, I stood under a soft rain, feeling a certain sense of catharsis. Memories that had just moments before felt asphyxiating lost much of their sting. But these fresh recollections from childhood felt like a tangled mess that needed to be sorted through, examined, and reconsidered. I would spend the next few months doing so in therapy and conversations with old friends. It didn't take long for a question that should have been obvious to emerge: Having managed to avoid being pulled directly into my country's war, why did I later volunteer to spend years working in war zones? Was there a through line?

∿∿ I wrote the email on a whim and felt a pang of regret seconds after hitting Send. It was the fall of 2006, and I was a little more than a year into a new job at the *Washington Post*, where I covered cops and courts in a suburban bureau in Maryland. I had a great editor, enjoyed covering a range of tragic and quirky crime cases, and was beginning to feel settled in Washington, DC. The newspaper's foreign desk was struggling to keep its large Baghdad bureau staffed as the invasion of Iraq had turned into a bloody quagmire, and editors had begun recruiting early career reporters for two-month stints in Baghdad. It was a high-profile and high-stakes assignment with a guaranteed path to front-page bylines. For some of my colleagues, Baghdad tours had led to full-time foreign correspondent jobs or promotions elsewhere in the newsroom. The first step was to get buy-in from my manager, who then put my name forward to the foreign editor. I half hoped they would thank me for raising my hand but turn me down for lack of experience. But with a civil war escalating, Baghdad coverage was a high priority, and the paper was running low on experienced conflict reporters to send. The day after I volunteered, everyone in the newsroom had signed off on my assignment, which would start in mid-January 2007.

To prepare, I was fitted for body armor and sent to a short hostile-reporting workshop in rural Virginia taught by British former soldiers who took great pleasure in executing a mock kidnapping exercise during which we were forced out of a van at gunpoint. I was so busy and anxious about the trip that I don't recall stopping to consider why I had volunteered and what I hoped it would lead to. I was given a stack of books to read, spent hours applying for a visa at the crumbling Iraqi embassy in Dupont Circle, and agonized about what to pack for my first overseas assignment.

I landed in the Iraqi capital one morning, nervous and severely jet-lagged, and followed the complicated instructions to find Omar, our affable bureau driver. I slipped into the front seat of the dilapidated bulletproof Mercedes-Benz and made the first of many rookie mistakes: I fastened my seat belt. Omar shook his head and ordered me to unclick it: in Iraq, he said, only a foreigner would wear a seat belt, and being visibly foreign in a city teeming with militia checkpoints was a sure way to get kidnapped. Omar drove frighteningly fast as we took a circuitous route to my new home. As a Sunni, he needed to avoid areas controlled by Shiite militias, I later learned. It had been a few weeks since Saddam Hussein had been executed in a grotesque, American-orchestrated affair. The city felt tense.

Minutes after walking into our bureau, a three-story house in a walled-off compound, before I had a chance to unpack, I was pulled into a mad scramble to report a breaking news story. A twenty-eight-year-old American woman who worked for the National Democratic Institute in Baghdad had been killed in a brazen daytime attack after leaving a meeting. I filed a story within a couple of hours and took satisfaction in typing the dateline in all caps: BAGHDAD. In the days that followed, there was a torrent of news to cover. The troop surge President George W. Bush had ordered was in full swing, and the American war effort was faltering. During my first weekend in town, I wrote about an attack on a provincial government building where a handful of lightly protected American soldiers were abducted at gunpoint and later executed. A dozen other American service members were killed in a helicopter crash. I slept little those first few days, leaning heavily on coffee to stay alert.

Car bombs and suicide bombings rattled the capital every day. Driving through the city, we'd see blast craters and blackened, disfigured buildings every other block. Checkpoints were manned by jumpy gunmen who kept their fingers on the triggers of AK-47s. The bureau security advisor requested that we keep in-person interviews to under fifteen minutes and that we never announce our plans beforehand, because the threat of kidnapping was extraordinarily high. At night, I learned to fall asleep listening to the low rumble of artillery the US military fired at suspected al-Qaeda hideouts in the outer bands of the capital. Sectarian bloodletting had become so widespread that several members of our staff were too scared to go to their neighborhoods at night. Some began sleeping on cots in the living room.

Because of the time difference, responding to editors in Washington kept us up late at night and meant we often worked eighteen-hour days. The American military, setting in motion a counterinsurgency strategy, was trying to drum up support for the war back home, which presented correspondents with numerous opportunities to fly around the country on daredevil helicopter rides with generals and to embed with combat units on the front lines.

Looking back on those heady weeks now makes my introduction to war reporting sound like a terrifying crucible—and it certainly was. But strangely, I don't recall feeling frightened. In important ways, my childhood in Colombia had conditioned me to navigate Iraq's maze of dangers. It may sound strange, but I look back on those weeks as perhaps the most fun and invigorating of my life. I was running high on adrenaline, which made me hypervigilant and hyperproductive. Editors at the highest levels of the paper were complimenting my work, which made me feel like I had entered the big leagues of journalism. The walled-off compound where we lived and worked was home to a small group of foreign correspondents and aid workers, many of them also young and ambitious. We partied at night as hard as we worked during the day.

In late March, I spent the final days of my temporary Baghdad assignment with an army unit that had been tasked with building a small outpost at an abandoned school on a street that was a fault line in the sectarian war. During a nighttime patrol to get a lay of the land, I watched a Bradley Fighting Vehicle driving slowly through darkened streets get struck by an armor-piercing roadside bomb that had become a major killer of American troops. There were a few seconds of stunned silence as everyone took stock and realized the munition had not pierced the vehicle. The soldiers inside were intact.

In the article I wrote about the embed, I quoted a twenty-eight-year-old army staff sergeant from Phoenix named Brian Mancini. This was not his first Iraq deployment; he was skeptical of his mission and sick of the war. "If I die in Iraq this time," he said, at least "I won't have to worry about coming back again." A few months later, in July, a roadside bomb disfigured Brian's face. He struggled for years with physical and mental wounds that didn't get better over the years. In 2017, he died by suicide, according to the *Arizona Republic*, which quoted his mother saying Brian had simply been in "too much pain."

〰〰 After a couple of weeks of vacation, I returned home to Washington. My job in sleepy Rockville, Maryland, which I'd loved until I went to Iraq, now seemed profoundly unstimulating. I felt irritable and depressed, desperately missing the camaraderie I had found among the wacky characters in the Baghdad press corps. But a cure to my malaise was at hand: senior editors soon asked if I would be interested in a permanent role in our Baghdad bureau. The answer was an immediate, emphatic *yes!* The prospect of jumping back into that cauldron of violence and adventure instantly lifted my mood. I didn't realize it then, but I was craving another sustained jolt of adrenaline. My employer would offer no shortage of them over the next few years.

I sold my car, put my belongings in storage, and returned to Baghdad in early 2008 for a yearlong assignment. Just a few years after graduating from college, I was a foreign correspondent at one of the world's most prestigious news organizations. At the time, war zone reporters at the *Post* typically took a month off for every month we were on duty. That schedule established an unhealthy cycle: periods of high stress, little sleep, and a crusading approach to work followed by a few weeks off, when it was often hard to distinguish between exhaustion and depression.

In Baghdad, almost every journalist at the time smoked heavily. I picked up the habit. Heavy drinking at night was the norm, even on weekdays—which, at the time, seemed like a reasonable coping mechanism in a violent, chaotic place. At the end of my first year, I readily signed up for a second year in Baghdad. The incentives of those jobs made it easy to get pulled into war coverage for years on end, without noticing the toll it was taking, said Lulu Garcia-Navarro, who was then a Baghdad-based correspondent for National Public Radio, and became a friend. "You're under life-threatening danger, and it's also a big story," she said. "The more you put yourself out there, the more you keep working, the more you get swept into this hero narrative."

My memories of the bloodiest days I witnessed in Iraq are spotty, but a handful have come roaring back during ayahuasca ceremonies. During a period of massive suicide bombings, I remember walking into the morgue of a hospital and seeing the charred bodies of several babies that had been laid on a table on cafeteria trays. Outside were women in black abayas, full-body garments, wailing as they slammed the dirt with their fists. I filed a quick draft of a story and got an email back from the editor thanking me and noting that he had "toned down the wailing widows."

In the summer of 2009, I spent several days with an army unit at a combat outpost in Sadr City run by a lieutenant colonel named Tim Karcher. He was funny and kind, and invited me to join him on all his meetings and missions. Days after I left, his legs were blown off. Tim survived.

The most scarring experience came in January 2010, when I was running the bureau in Baghdad, which we shared with NPR. On a routine workday, I had gone to the Green Zone to interview the Iraqi government spokesman about useless handheld bomb-detection devices Iraq had spent a fortune on. The interview came to an abrupt halt as a series of blasts thundered nearby, followed by a hail of bullets. En route to the bureau, where I assumed I'd have to soon write yet another bombing story, I learned that our compound had been among the targets attacked that day. Lulu had arrived in Baghdad that morning, and she was in the shower when the blast left half of our house in ruins. Because the bombing had been preceded by a gunfight at the gate of our complex, most of our employees had taken refuge in the bureau's so-called safe room, a windowless pantry outfitted with bottles of water, canned food, buckets to pee in, and the phone numbers of the US military in Iraq.

When I arrived home, I found two of our Iraqi employees who had not managed to get to the pantry in time bleeding from the head. My laptop had been flung from the desk where I had been working early that morning. Its screen had shattered against a wall. Lulu and my *Washington Post* colleague Leila Fadel, who later became an NPR host, were working maniacally. I saw Lulu standing by the giant smoldering crater outside our house describing the gory scene on a satellite phone, looking wild-eyed and disheveled. Leila looked upset that she couldn't find a cable to copy photos from a digital camera onto a computer. I emailed the editors to tell them what had happened and assured them we'd file a story as quickly as possible.

Soon, it dawned on us that the priority needed to be to get our wounded colleagues medical care. The roads leading to our compound had been barricaded, as often happened after bombings, to avoid a second strike. None of us had medical training. The only idea I came up with at the time was to call a gynecologist I had gone out on a couple of dates with in Washington, where it was about 4:00 a.m. Jolted awake, the doctor told me to put light pressure on the wounds with bandages, to check if their pupils could follow a moving finger, and to keep them awake and talking. Thankfully, they recovered. That night, Leila and I squatted at the home of a British journalist, who took us in for several days. We drank heavily, cried, and walked around in a daze during the next couple of weeks.

After nearly two years, I had been offered a new assignment in the region, which meant my time in Iraq was coming to a close. My final tasks included finding a new house for the bureau and laying off several Iraqi colleagues, including one who had been injured in the blast. The sadness and sense of betrayal in their eyes was gutting. But it made business sense. Our operation in Iraq had grown when Iraq was a top story. Now, US troops were drawing down there as attention, resources, and firepower were shifting to Afghanistan, where the Obama administration had ordered a troop surge. Iraq, a war the United States did not quite lose but certainly did not win, was limping to an untidy conclusion. Washington set its sights on the fight against the Taliban, a war that had always been more defensible, politically and morally.

I would be part of that shift. The editors offered me a new assignment based in Cairo as a roving correspondent tasked with filling in at our bureau in Afghanistan every couple of months. Soon after I settled into that position, the Arab Spring kicked off, sparking a series of revolts and armed conflicts that kept me in a state of whiplash for the next two years. Toward the end of that period, I no longer drew satisfaction from periods of high stress and adrenaline. I took risks in the field more out of habit than the sense of duty that had propelled me earlier in my time overseas. I was often irritable, depressed, and profoundly lonely. In that vulnerable state, I entered into an ill-advised yearlong relationship. When it ended, I felt utterly heartbroken, lost, and adrift.

As a reward for my years in war zones, I was offered a high-profile assignment: Pentagon correspondent. I returned to Washington in the fall of 2012, ready to wean myself off the roller-coaster life of a war correspondent.

Few people seemed to notice at the time, but I was emotionally dysregulated. This was easy to hide from colleagues but became apparent to those who tried to form romantic bonds with me. A promising relationship with a British diplomat ended because I was often cold and prone to picking needless fights. I never felt entitled to PTSD as a diagnosis, but looking back now, it's clear I met some of the criteria and would have likely benefited from getting help. Being in crowded spaces like a packed subway car filled me with dread as I imagined how an explosion would play out. One day, when I was skiing, a controlled avalanche blast made me fall to my knees, paralyzed with fear, even though I understood I was in no danger.

I am convinced that my editors at the time would have been

empathetic and supportive had I confided I was struggling. But among correspondents who cover war and other traumatic events, there was a deeply rooted and widely shared fear that being unwell would limit career options. There were plenty of cautionary tales of colleagues whose names became associated with that dreaded four-letter diagnosis—PTSD. They were no longer in the game. Reaching out for help would have meant undermining my reputation as a re-silient and stoic professional, which had become a pillar of my sense of self. I said nothing. Reputation intact, after two years covering the Pentagon, I got an unexpected email from the deputy Opinion editor at the *New York Times*, who offered me a job on the newspaper's edi-torial board. Once again, I jumped at the opportunity. The job gave me the chance to opine on foreign policy and armed conflict without having to see it up close. I made an early splash in the role.

But I now realize that suppressing symptoms of unprocessed trauma does not make it go away. And one day, the coping mechanisms stop working.

〰〰 The toll of war was the furthest thing on my mind when I un-raveled in Brazil in 2017. But soon after I began turning to aya-huasca as a tool for introspection and healing, flashbacks from the war of my childhood and the ones I covered as an adult began sur-facing. I never went into a ceremony with the intention to dive into those chapters of the past. But ayahuasca often seems more prone to hand out assignments rather than to accept requests. So I found myself assembling a messy mosaic of wartime memories. Many of these scenes and flashbacks grabbed me with breathtaking tenac-ity and focus. Once I had latched onto one, it was impossible to shift to a new thought until I had given the recollection lengthy consideration and surrendered to the emotions it stirred. I came to see these wartime scenes and memories as cases being pursued by tiny, indignant litigants who had been waiting for their day in court in some dark, stuffy recess of my brain. The way psychoactive substances like ayahuasca affect memory retrieval and reconsideration remains poorly understood, said Manoj Dass, a cognitive neuropsychopharmacologist at Johns Hopkins University who studies the correlation between memory and drug use. He told me there is no hard evidence that ayahuasca and substances like it unveil repressed memories. Indeed, he suspects psychedelics can sometimes create distorted or false memories. But Manoj said there is growing evidence that psychedelics, by sparking periods of disruptive thinking, create an opportunity to "reconsolidate" memories. In practice, he said, that means gaining the ability to reassemble a set of facts in a way that fundamentally shifts how you understand them and how they make you feel. Obsessive, recurring thoughts—which depressed and traumatized people often struggle with—can suddenly become elements of a clearer narrative, which loosens their grip.

"Reconsolidation is like changing the way the memory was initially encoded," he said. "It seems like it's meant to be an adaptive process where, okay, it's good to remember these negative things, but you don't need to remember them detail for detail."

Over the years, as my recollections of war multiplied, I began seeing the outlines of a narrative of my life that made a lot of sense. This required sitting with difficult, often uncomfortable questions that I had long ignored. How scarring had it been to grow up in a country at war? How much guilt is appropriate for having dodged my legal duty to serve in uniform as a teenager? Why the hell had I volunteered to cover wars—and stuck with it so long? Was there a clear link to be drawn between the conflicts I fled and the ones I later volunteered to barrel into?

I now have answers to those questions, some tentative, some painfully obvious. Growing up in Colombia in the 1980s and 1990s was profoundly traumatic. It's the reason I'm among the more than 9 percent of Colombians who live abroad. To be uprooted from one's homeland, even under privileged circumstances, is to go through life with a wound that never quite heals. Ever since I left, the first notes of the Colombian national anthem unfailingly make tears pool in my eyes. I used to be perplexed and embarrassed by that reaction. Now

I embrace it as a tiny ritual of mourning that honors the fact that some of us go through life feeling forever a little adrift, never quite at home anywhere.

I hate that having dodged military service by paying a bribe is part of my story. It was dishonorable. It was wrong. I hate that I could do it while so many had no choice. It added to the torrent of transgressions, big and small, that keep a society in a state of perpetual war. As I contemplated that act, initially with enormous guilt and shame, I found myself wondering if those feelings had been part of what propelled me to spend years in war zones. I clearly left Colombia with a sense of unfinished business and a need to atone, somewhere, somehow. Regardless of how dominant a role it played in my decision to work in war zones, this much is clear: I have gained the ability to look back on these younger versions of myself with greater compassion. That has made these chapters of my life easier to carry, to speak about, and to explain to myself and others.

13　A KETAMINE "FIELD TRIP"

THE PSYCHEDELICS CONFERENCE IN MIAMI was fittingly called Wonderland. The organizers hailed the November 2022 symposium as the largest gathering to date of "visionaries and pioneers" united in a bold quest to reimagine the "future of psychedelic medicine, the business of mental health, and the future of longevity medicine."

The trade floor booths at the large convention center brimmed with colorful characters and exhibits that quickly led to sensory overload. A young woman hawked a virtual reality set that promised to catalyze psychedelic trip insights. A music player wired to mushrooms was said to turn fungal wisdom into melody. And a company called Liquid IV Therapy—which had no discernible link to psychedelics—offered $245 injections of vitamins and minerals to treat the hangovers of those who overindulged at the nightly after-parties. Tucked all the way in the back of the space was a translucent dome that served as a space for Indigenous music and rituals.

I spent three days shifting between two stages where a dizzying array of quacks, showboats, and acclaimed scientists took turns holding court. The attendees seemed more riveted by hyperbolic claims and rants about the war on drugs than lessons about neuroscience or the regulatory hurdles standing in the way of lawfully prescribing psychoactive drugs.

Several names on the program caught my attention. There was Mike Zapolin, an entrepreneur who goes by "Zappy" and non-ironically uses the title "Psychedelic Concierge to the Stars." The German investor Christian Angermayer, a leading funder of psychedelic ventures, spoke fervently about a not-too-distant future in which humans could opt out of aging. Rick Doblin, the founder of the Multidisciplinary Association for Psychedelic Studies, the leading organization paving the way for the lawful use of psychedelics in medicine, dared attendees to dream big.

"We want to work toward a world of net-zero trauma by 2070," he thundered.

I had come to Wonderland expecting the nuttiness, craven capitalism, and bedazzlement that have come to define the so-called psychedelic renaissance. But my primary motivation was to sit down with some of the top academics in the field to understand what makes them optimistic—and what gives them pause.

Given all I had seen and experienced in the Wild West of retreats and spiritual communities over the past year, I wanted to get a glimpse of the emerging clinical model, which offered a more regimented and secular approach to psychedelic healing.

There has been a solidifying consensus among psychiatrists that psychedelics may revolutionize mental health treatment. A key source of optimism was a pair of bureaucratic moves by the Food and Drug Administration. In 2017, federal regulators designated MDMA, the drug known as ecstasy, as a "breakthrough therapy" to treat post-traumatic stress disorder. That label is given to drugs that appear to outperform conventional therapies in clinical trials and is meant to accelerate research that brings them to market. The following year, the agency granted psilocybin the same designation based on studies showing its efficacy to treat depression.

In a field that has seen no major breakthroughs since the advent of antidepressants in the 1980s, this was cause for celebration. But vexing questions about the future of the field remain unanswered.

Will the encouraging results scientists have seen in clinical trials hold up when and if these substances become broadly available to patients? After all, there's been a self-selecting dynamic to the kind of scientists and patients who have been drawn to psychedelic studies.

If the clinical setting lacks the spiritual and mystical dimension that is so central to these experiences in retreats and religious circles, would something crucial be lost? Are there patients with underlying conditions—such as propensity for schizophrenia—for whom psychedelic trips might be more destabilizing than healing? Just how vital is the role of psychotherapy in harnessing the healing potential of mind-bending sessions? And if these therapies become available in our health care system, will their cost be prohibitive?

After spending hours interviewing some of the leading scholars shaping this field, I was struck by how much remains up in the air. Most expressed concern that the hype is outpacing the science.

Dr. Christopher Pittenger, a psychiatrist who leads Yale University's Program for Psychedelic Science, told me that through brain-imaging technology, scientists have discovered that compounds like DMT and psilocybin lead neurons to grow new synapses. Practically speaking, that means the wiring linking various components of the brain gets a reset.

"We know they do interesting things while people are intoxicated to the way different brain circuits are organized relative to one another," he said. "And we know that a large fraction of people who are using these substances under particular circumstances get symptom improvement."

But the correlation between the two remains a mystery. "There's an enormous amount we don't know," he said.

Dr. Natalie Gukasyan, a psychiatrist at Johns Hopkins University who has given psilocybin to patients with anorexia, said that psychedelic trips appear to generate a period of enhanced "cognitive flexibility." For people who have been in the grip of obsessive or fatalistic thought loops, that can generate a "window of opportunity that can allow people to make substantive changes in their patterns of thinking and behavior," she said. "Your entire worldview can change."

But can that be explained solely by changes in brain activity? Or is the mystical experience—which can't be captured or measured in brain scans—essential? "I don't think there's a unified idea of why this is so powerful," she told me.

One major obstacle has been the challenge of doing placebo-controlled clinical trials with psychedelics—the gold standard for determining whether new drugs or interventions are effective. After all, psychedelic study participants can generally detect whether they're in the placebo group.

Dr. Michael P. Bogenschutz, a psychiatrist who leads the Langone Center for Psychedelic Medicine at New York University, told me he worries that the preliminary results of highly controlled clinical trials are creating the impression that psychedelic trips are inherently healing.

They may well prove to be powerful tools to shift cognition and behavior, he argued, but without strong safeguards and solid ethics, the field will be ripe for abusive and predatory behavior.

"I think it's very dangerous to think that these substances are innocuous just because people don't die of an overdose or become addicted," he said. "People are in a remarkably vulnerable state during these experiences."

〰〰 Janis Phelps, a psychologist and professor at the California Institute of Integral Studies, has given that concern a lot of thought. It's what prompted her in 2016 to launch the first academic certificate program for psychedelic therapists in the United States. Early in her career, Janis briefly dabbled in MDMA-assisted therapy, giving patients the drug known as ecstasy to help them open up during psychotherapy. It was a short-lived modality; in 1985, the DEA added MDMA to its list of banned narcotics.

A few years later, Janis traveled to the Peruvian Amazon to drink ayahuasca with Indigenous healers, an experience that filled her with wonder. "It laid me on my rear," she told me, noting she meant that literally and figuratively.

Those sessions informed her understanding of the role substance-induced altered states of consciousness can play in therapy. Janis marveled at how much a person could intuit and change in a short period of time. As if by divine intervention, "your inner eye is turned inward into a place beyond your ego," she said.

For most of her career, the idea of mixing banned drugs with therapy was a nonstarter. But by 2016, Janis saw an opening. Many people in her field were feeling stuck, she said. A new wave of psychedelic studies carried out by reputable scientists was resurrecting a field of research hastily shut down in the 1970s by the Nixon administration's war on drugs.

The cohort that signed up for the inaugural training was small. The program was open only to doctors and licensed mental health care professionals, some of whom asked that their involvement remain private, for fear that it could harm their reputations and future job prospects. Among them was a seasoned psychiatrist who told Janis he had lost faith in the go-to intervention for depression.

"I've been in an existential dilemma as a psychiatrist because I'm pained every time I write another script for Prozac or Zoloft," Janis recalled the man saying. "I know it's numbing out their symptoms, but it's not getting to the heart of the matter."

Years of clinical practice have led Janis to believe that the most substantive type of healing happens when patients find the tools and wherewithal to do profound introspection. The best therapists have mastered the art of being a "midwife for that work," Janis said, steering patients gently as they discover what has been at the root of their distress and what they can do about it.

"The best thing that humans can do for one another is not to fill their hearts and minds with information that one human feels is important," Janis said. "Rather, it's drawing out the wisdom in someone else."

Patients who are in the grip of trauma or depression are often not in a position to do that. But psychedelics, when administered in a safe and controlled setting, can create extraordinary windows of opportunity, Janis said. When we spoke in early 2023, more than eight hundred health professionals had gone through her training. Several competitors had launched similar programs, catering to a surge of therapists who had begun or aspired to work with psychedelics.

Those working legally had started giving patients ketamine, an anesthetic that can be prescribed off-label for treatment of psychiatric conditions. At low doses, it induces a dissociative, psychedelic-like state. Others had begun offering retreats abroad or offered to help people make sense of self-guided psychedelic trips. Some had given up professional licenses and reinvented themselves as "coaches" in order to guide psychedelic experiences.

Though she arguably played a leading role in destigmatizing psychedelic therapy, Janis told me she felt uneasy about how quickly the field was growing and how unwieldy it had become. Some of its pioneers, predictably, were risk-takers, the kind of people prone to cutting corners and crossing boundaries. The bombastic claims about psychedelics that had become common in the press and promotional material were setting people up for disappointment, or worse, Janis feared. "There's no magic bullet," she said.

〜〜〜 I wasn't expecting magic, per se, when I walked into the San Diego ketamine clinic that November. But it would be a lie to say the marketing for Field Trip, one of the pioneering brick-and-mortar psychedelic therapy businesses, didn't have the intended effect on me.

The check-in process felt more like arriving at a bougie spa than a medical appointment. The walls were decorated with faux greenery. Golden lamps dangled from the lobby's high ceiling. Plants and crystals gave the waiting room, which featured modern white lounge chairs and a green sofa covered in fluffy cushions, feng shui vibes. The receptionist handed me a pair of fuzzy gray socks, the kind you get in a business-class-flight amenity kit, and pointed to a menu from which I was to select snacks to enjoy after my treatment. I picked mixed nuts, a fruit plate, and mushroom tea.

Then Lauren Cabaldon, the psychotherapist who would be overseeing my treatment, appeared, flashing a radiant smile. "Welcome to Field Trip," she said before guiding me to a small treatment room with a white zero-gravity reclining chair. That's where I would soon get an intramuscular injection of ketamine from a nurse whose streaks of pink hair felt very much on brand.

I began contemplating doing a ketamine session at one of Field Trip's clinics after interviewing Ronan Levy, one of the company's founders, in the summer of 2022. The conversation with Ronan, a Canadian attorney who had previously worked in the medical cannabis business, left me feeling at once intrigued and skeptical. The company, which raised millions from venture capitalists, went public in October 2020, among the first of dozens of start-ups that saw in the nation's mental health crisis a huge business opportunity.

Ketamine was produced in the 1960s by drug developers seeking to create an anesthetic with fewer side effects. It became widely used as a sedative in veterinary and human medicine over the decades, but there was no inkling the drug could treat mental health conditions until the 1990s. Researchers at Yale University discovered that ketamine provided some people with depression immediate relief, making it a potential game changer in psychiatry. The most widely used drugs for depression, selective serotonin reuptake inhibitors, or SSRIs, don't work for many patients and often take weeks to start having an effect. Many people who take them experience significant side effects, including weight gain and a lower sex drive.

Clinicians at Yale and other institutions began administering ketamine to some patients off-label. But they cautioned that the drug should be used judiciously, and only after conventional options had been exhausted. After all, there was limited information about the long-term efficacy and safety of ketamine in mental health treatment.

Had ketamine been a new drug, pharmaceutical companies would have had a strong incentive to fund the kind of robust clinical trials federal regulators would have required to approve its use as a treatment for depression.

But ketamine's patent expired in 2002, which meant there was little to gain by bankrolling years of costly research.

The absence of a more solid scientific and regulatory foundation did not stop ketamine from emerging as a strongly hyped and aggressively marketed psychiatric drug starting around 2018.

Companies like Field Trip, which is based in Toronto, saw in ketamine an opportunity to establish brand recognition and a treatment model they hoped would soon incorporate MDMA and psychoactive mushrooms.

By the time I spoke to Ronan, his company had raised some $96 million and was operating nine clinics in Canada and the United States. He outlined a grand vision. In addition to its clinics, Field Trip was developing a novel psychedelic compound called FT-104, which was structurally similar to psilocybin but had the potential to become a patentable and revenue-generating drug. The company was also growing psilocybin mushrooms in Jamaica, where they are legal, with the intention of becoming a leading supplier when the regulatory landscape became more permissive.

If all went according to plan, Ronan told me, he aspired to open more than seventy clinics that he hoped would radically transform how people thought about mental health. He had been pondering how CrossFit became such a disruptive force in fitness, and was keen to emulate that brand's success. The mental health care system currently caters mainly to people who are unwell, Ronan noted. But psychedelics had the potential to do much more than alleviate suffering. They stood to turbocharge the outlook, mindset, and creative potential of people who were not exactly in distress but not quite thriving.

"I want Field Trip to be a lifestyle company and not a medical company," Ronan told me. "My ambition is to help people consciously, safely, and responsibly open up to a new world of possibilities through psychedelics."

〰〰 Psychedelics, one could argue, had helped unleash a world of new possibilities for me over the past year. In mid-2021, I told my editors that I was ready to wrap up my time in Brazil after more than four years of covering a torrent of bad news. My tour began as the country was in the throes of a brutal recession and a surge of violent crime, factors that led to the election of a divisive far-right president. Then came COVID, which took a devastating toll on Brazil. I was burned out and craved a change. Starting in early 2022, the newspaper agreed to let me spend a year working on this book, with institutional support.

By then, I had been dating Steve, the veterinary professor living in Minnesota, for just over seven months. He had managed to work remotely from Brazil during much of that time, which made clear we were quite compatible. But my looming departure from Brazil forced us to confront a big decision: whether we were ready to move in together. Laying down roots in the Midwest could have limited my job options once the book was done. But for the first time in my life, I chose to prioritize love over career prospects.

It was a leap of faith and it didn't take long before I started to question the wisdom of trading summertime in Brazil for the bone-chilling winter of Minnesota. My unease was reflected in Hugo's eyes the first few times I took him for walks outside our new home in Saint Paul in minus-ten-degree weather. *What on earth were you thinking, human?* his anguished eyes seemed to convey, paws burrowed in three inches of snow.

I had anticipated that spending a year chronicling the psychedelics world would be the most fun I would ever have as a journalist. But it soon became apparent the endeavor would be quite hard and emotionally taxing. Attending retreats as a reporter felt like sleeping with one eye open. I was constantly monitoring what was happening around me, making a mental note of which strands would contribute to a narrative. Naturally, that limited my ability to surrender to the mystery of these experiences, which is how insights arise and old wounds are tended.

In between reporting trips, my days were spent poring over the hundreds of interview transcripts and writing in fits and starts. Working on a book is a solitary task, and I had spent countless hours interviewing people about their depression, traumas, and suicidal ideation. I often walked away from the keyboard feeling drained and depressed. During periods of writing block, I fretted about my future. By writing this book, I had attached two loaded words to my professional brand: *depression* and *psychedelics*. Some days, it felt like a colossal mistake.

As a result of the research I had been doing, my social media feeds were flooded with ads for psychedelic retreats and ketamine clinics. Initially, I had intended to limit my personal participation as part of book research to ayahuasca ceremonies. But suddenly, a torrent of dreamy ketamine ads the algorithms were throwing my way proved quite seductive at a moment when I was particularly susceptible.

"Bring back 'the Happy.' Fast!" a Colorado company enticed. A competitor's Instagram post featured a placid-looking woman enjoying a hot drink in a sun-drenched room. "Ketamine *helped* my brain switch channels," the ad proclaimed.

Switch the channel! That's precisely what I need, I thought. I didn't need to ask my doctor. Clearly, ketamine was right for me!

During my conversation with Ronan, I had expressed interest in visiting one of their clinics to see how this one-on-one model worked. Field Trip put me in touch with Lauren, the lead clinician at the San Diego branch, one of the newest. When I followed up with Lauren in the fall, I was feeling particularly low and found myself asking how much it would cost to try a session as a patient. Field Trip generally recommended packages of five to six infusions, which cost upward of $5,000. A one-off would be $750, which would include brief psychotherapy sessions before and after the "medicine journey," as she called it. I made an appointment for early November. We agreed that this would be both a real therapeutic intervention and a journalistic exploration.

〰〰 During our introductory psychotherapy session on a video call, which took place the morning before my ketamine treatment, Lauren asked what I hoped to get from the experience. I told her I had been giving fear too much oxygen, allowing it to dominate my thinking and zap my creativity. I told her I wanted to learn how to cultivate faith—in myself, in the choices I had made, and in my ability to be at ease with uncertainty.

I surprised myself by telling Lauren something else: I had been carrying a lot of anger toward my mother in the wake of my father's death. Perhaps there would be room to explore those feelings. She listened with warmth and told me she looked forward to guiding my session in a few hours.

That afternoon, Lauren draped a white weighted blanket over me as I sank into the zero-gravity chair. It felt warm and nurturing. New age music played softly. I was provided a set of noise-canceling headphones and an eye mask with robust padding. The nurse would soon come in to inject eighty-five milligrams of ketamine into my right biceps. But first, Lauren read what she called "preflight instructions."

Speaking slowly and confidently, she assured me I would be safe and cared for throughout. "Trust the process, trust the medicine, and trust your inner healing intelligence," Lauren said. "Approach this journey with the curiosity of a beginner's mind."

She urged me to be fearless in exploring any visual or emotional realms I encountered. "If you see doors, open them," Lauren prodded. "If you see staircases, climb them; if you see bodies of water, go into them. Say yes to *everything*."

Frightening sights could be instructive too, she said. "Inquire about it and lean into it," she urged. "Part of the healing comes from approaching that which is uncomfortable or even disturbing."

When she reached the end of the script, Lauren asked me to set an intention. My heart raced as I let out a big sigh. "I'd like to strengthen my faith," I said barely above a whisper. Saying it felt like a prayer, and I allowed myself to hope it would be answered.

Shortly after I put on the headphones and covered my eyes, the nurse walked into the room. As Lauren tapped a gong, I felt the pinch of the needle and a slight burning sensation as the ketamine seeped into my muscle and wandered through my veins. Within a minute, I felt a blissful withdrawal. My ability to think dissolved. This was radically different from the altered states I had experienced on aya-huasca. On ketamine, I retained strong powers of perception, but lost any sense of being in a body with limbs that can move at will. Gone too was my ability to think coherent thoughts, the type that can be put into words. I felt like a soul, weightless and shapeless, drifting into a kaleidoscope of black-and-white shapes that drew me in, working in perfect harmony with the playlist Lauren had curated especially for me.

Some forty-five minutes after the injection, my thinking mind snapped back on. *Fear and faith*, I suddenly thought with wonder. Those two monosyllabic terms are states locked in a perpetual dance. On matters mundane and existential, we listen to both, hoping to strike the right balance. It dawned on me I had been keeping faith on the shortest of leashes, while fear, unruly and insatiable, thrashed around without restraint. In my ketamine-altered state, this dichotomy felt revelatory and clarifying, like a password that had suddenly unlocked a door I had been trying to kick open for days. Faith and fear. I took stock of people who had shown faith in me, personally and professionally, which led to a recalibration. I loosened my grip on faith while gently reeling fear in. I considered how much anguish I had come to feel about how future employers would think of the mental health challenges I disclose in this book. It was a legitimate fear, for sure. But I suddenly realized some might give more weight to the perspective and resilience they have yielded. Have faith.

Suddenly, the smell of palo santo, which Lauren burns to signal that a session is drawing to a close, snapped me back into the present moment. I was reluctant to take off my mask and exit this dreamy state.

"You had quite a journey," Lauren said as my eyes adjusted to the light. I had been out for an hour and ten minutes, she said. I confessed I had begun to fear—that word again!—that I was over-staying my welcome. I hadn't, Lauren assured me. She suggested I explore that concern and asked whether sensing that I was taking up space and people's time was something I struggle with. Yes, I said, I had always been hypervigilant about how I was being perceived and whether I was annoying or inconveniencing people.

"Does that come from your mother?" she asked.

The question caught me off guard, but she was onto something. My mother had never been good with boundaries. When she erupted in fits of rage or became absorbed in paranoid delusions, it never seemed to register how she was being perceived.

"She could be a bit of a bulldozer," I told Lauren. "I wonder if that is why I became so afraid of repeating those patterns and not noticing."

"You've been overcorrecting," she offered.

Lauren asked how that fear had shaped the way I approach rela-tionships. I told her it made me predisposed to distrust people and to place a high premium on self-sufficiency. "People who are nour-ishing one day can turn into the devil the next," I said, slurring my words a bit as the effects of the drug abated.

"You had to learn that to survive," she said. "But is that pattern serving you now?"

We both knew the answer.

Patterns that have formed over years take time to override, Lauren said. Seeing them is the first step. "It's a process of deep unlearning, and that doesn't happen overnight."

I left the clinic late that afternoon feeling a deep sense of calm. I wouldn't say the session changed the channel. But it certainly wiped out a lot of static.

That night, I pondered my feelings toward my mother, from whom I've been largely estranged most of my adult life. It's a sore subject I tend to avoid thinking about unless something forces my hand. One such event was my father's death in October 2020. While my parents had long been divorced, my mom became a caretaker as cancer ravaged her former spouse. Watching her in that role had reminded me of a tender side that defined our bond when I was a child. Memories of that gentle, nourishing mother had been largely drowned out by memories of the tumultuous years after their marriage came undone. For better or for worse, those had become the defining memories of my childhood.

As I cleaned out my father's bedroom the day after he died, I stumbled onto a pile of old letters and legal filings from the tumultuous era that followed their divorce.

Several were long, rambling letters my mother had written—to my father, to me, to other relatives. They included wild, hurtful, and mostly unfounded accusations. One she penned after I came out of the closet at nineteen was particularly scornful. It used a slur, *maricón*, the Spanish word for "faggot."

Reeling from the loss of my father, I felt compelled to salvage all those documents. It felt worthwhile to preserve a record of those turbulent years. The fading ink on yellowing pieces of paper was evidence of how destabilizing that era had been. They helped explain why I had flown so far from the nest, why I spent so much of my life in fight-or-flight mode. They vindicated my decision to keep my mother at arm's length, a choice that has never ceased causing me pain. Perhaps, I thought then, one day I would have the emotional wherewithal to go over them carefully. Maybe I would eventually share them with my sisters, and we could jointly make sense of a period we seldom discuss.

I kept the documents, perhaps three hundred pages in all, inside a tote bag we got from the funeral home where my father's body was cremated, the same one that briefly contained his ashes.

After scattering his remains during a brief ceremony marred by rain, I took the papers to Brazil, and later to Minnesota, figuring that eventually I would have the time and headspace to make sense of their content.

The night after taking ketamine, I changed my mind. It suddenly became clear to me that I was well acquainted enough with the documents and what they conveyed. There was no compelling reason to continue holding on to these tokens of pain and anger. I resolved to burn them, to feed them to a roaring bonfire on a starry night. Turning those pages into ashes may not be the key to closure or forgiveness. But it became clear to me that it would be a worthwhile ritual to bring me a step closer to letting a painful chapter of the past be in the past.

〰〰 A few months after my ketamine journey, a jarring email landed in my inbox. It informed Field Trip patients that the company was winding down operations. Having burned through the capital it raised, Field Trip had failed to build a sustainable business model. The marketplace, it had become clear, was not ready for a psychedelic CrossFit.

I called Lauren and asked her for a postmortem. During her time at Field Trip, she saw extraordinary outcomes, including people who managed to wean themselves off antidepressants and make the kind of breakthroughs that are often unattainable merely through talk therapy. But very few people could afford to pay some $5,000 out of pocket for a package of sessions, and very few insurance providers cover ketamine therapy. "It makes it inaccessible to a large portion of the population," Lauren said.

After losing her job, Lauren found a new role as director of training at a nonprofit start-up called Fireside Project, a hotline that caters to people who are experiencing distressing psychedelic trips at home. It's staffed by volunteers, who are not necessarily clinically trained. For now, Lauren said, it felt like a place where she could have the biggest impact. "There are so many people out there who are self-medicating and trying to come off SSRIs with these medicines," she told me. "And they often do need some sort of guide and support."

Soon, I would meet a pair of researchers employed by the federal government who got permission to create a proof of concept for psychedelic therapy in a conservative and risk-averse bureaucracy: the Department of Veterans Affairs.

14 "WRECKING BALL"

MDMA as Medicine at a VA Hospital

CHRIS CONLOGUE ARRIVED THIRTY MINUTES early for his appointment at the Veterans Affairs hospital in Loma Linda, California. His heart thumped. Walking toward the entrance of the sprawling tan-colored medical center, every step was a struggle, "like I was wearing lead boots," the army veteran recalled of that morning in early December 2021. "I was calmer in the middle of combat than I was going into that."

Chris had been coming to the Loma Linda VA regularly since 2018, when doctors there gave him a grim diagnosis. At thirty-four, he was on the brink of irreversible liver failure from years of binge drinking.

A team of specialists at the government medical center had persuaded Chris to enroll in an inpatient program for alcohol abuse. They cared for him during the agony of withdrawal, which made him hallucinate and spasm for days.

Once he was sober, a clinician suggested that Chris take the diagnostic test for post-traumatic stress disorder. Despite having served in Iraq during the first months of the war, Chris had never felt entitled to the PTSD label. But the test showed he fully met the criteria.

To treat his symptoms, which included insomnia, recurring night-mares, and hypervigilance, therapists at the VA prescribed Chris an antidepressant, administered cognitive behavioral therapy, and taught him how to meditate. He was grateful for those tools, which helped stabilize his mood somewhat. But Chris was still in distress.

In early 2021, one of the clinicians who had helped Chris get sober raised a possibility that astonished him. Dr. Allie Kaigle, a specialist in substance use disorders, told Chris the VA was recruiting patients for a groundbreaking study using MDMA, the drug known as ec-stasy, as a treatment for PTSD. The theory, she explained, was that the mind-altering drug, in conjunction with intense psychotherapy over the course of a few weeks, could address the root causes of trauma. Chris met the criteria for the study, the first of a handful of clinical trials conducted at Veterans Affairs hospitals around the country using psychedelics.

The Drug Enforcement Administration lists MDMA in its top tier of dangerous drugs, a designation reserved for substances with a high potential for abuse and no proven medical use. Yet the very VA clinicians who had ably helped him get sober were now raising the possibility of taking an unlawful drug, on government premises, and calling it therapy.

The clinical trial he was invited to join marked the first time the federal government administered psychedelics as part of authorized clinical studies since a promising wave of research came to a screech-ing halt when President Nixon declared a war on drugs in the 1970s.

To be eligible, Chris would have to agree to stop taking antide-pressants. He would also have to sign a lengthy consent form that underscored the experimental nature of the therapy and listed sev-eral possible risks. MDMA could make him irritable and anxious for a few days, worsen his insomnia, and possibly darken his mood. His sole psychedelic experience, a mushroom trip many years ago, had been terrifying. As he pondered whether to join the study, a vision crystallized in his mind. Chris told me he saw himself facing the Hoover Dam with a finger plugging a leak. Behind the wall was a torrent of sorrow and distress that had built up for years. He didn't know much about psychedelics, but Chris came to understand what he was invited to do as a radical measure.

Taking MDMA in a therapeutic setting, he intuited, would amount to taking "a freaking sledgehammer" to the dam. The thought was both terrifying and exhilarating. The whole thing felt like a huge gamble. Would this drug be the key to pacifying his unbearable mind, or might it further untether him? After tossing and turning over it for days, he was in.

〰 The MDMA trial at the Loma Linda VA may not have happened had it not been for an odd encounter in 2010 at the library of the Medical College of Georgia. Shannon Remick, then a first-year medical student, was picking up her textbooks for the semester when a librarian who had a bit of a hippie streak handed her a paperback and suggested she buy it.

The book was *Food of the Gods: The Search for the Original Tree of Knowledge,* by the American ethnobotanist Terence McKenna, who played a leading role in reviving interest in the history of psychedelics used in spiritual and therapeutic settings.

Shannon devoured McKenna's book, which traces how mind-altering drugs have shaped culture, spirituality, and health for millennia. The 1992 book puts forward the "Stoned Ape Theory," an unproven and widely doubted hypothesis suggesting that psilocybin mushrooms may have given our hominid ancestors a major cognitive leap thousands of years ago by enhancing their ability to think strategically and collaborate.

McKenna criticizes the blanket prohibition on drugs, lamenting that it cut off lawful access to compounds humans had long relied on to "experience personally the transcendental and the sacred." Drug laws, McKenna argued, deprived modern humans of a powerful tool that had helped our ancestors maintain a "symbiotic relationship to the earth."

Those ideas resonated powerfully for Shannon, the daughter of military veterans, who was raised on a farm in Georgia. They made her reconsider something mysterious that happened one night in 2008, when she returned home exhausted after taking the Medical College Admission Test. Despite months of studying, Shannon was convinced she had flunked. She felt like an utter failure, academically and personally, someone so worthless that she "might as well be dead," Shannon told me.

That night, along with a handful of friends who came to her place, Shannon took MDMA for the first time. Within minutes, those dark thoughts that had been swelling in her mind for months evaporated. They were replaced by an overwhelming sense of love and self-compassion. Shannon was astonished. It was like this tiny pill had changed the channel in her mind from a horror show to a blissful scene.

"It was just unbelievable, to go from that low of not wanting to be alive to being so grateful that I have a body that keeps me alive," she recalled. This altered state of mind had allowed Shannon to zoom out of the minutiae that can make everyday existence feel uncertain and unbearable, and left her with a panoramic view that was comforting. It may sound corny, she acknowledged, but the core truth she was left with that night was this: through good times and bad, we retain the capacity to love and to be loved. That makes staying alive worthwhile. With love, she said, "we can weather the storms."

Shannon's fears about having failed the MCAT proved unfounded; she passed with flying colors. The MDMA-induced turnaround she experienced that night felt nothing short of miraculous. After reading the book, Shannon began to think of the drug as medicinal. A few years into medical school, she decided to explore that idea more deeply in a research paper for a class on the history of medicine.

Titled "Psychedelics and Psychiatry: A Brief Look at the Past and the Present," the paper traced the convoluted history of government research into psychedelics. It included promising efforts to use LSD to treat alcoholism—including at a Veterans Affairs hospital in Kansas in the 1960s—and a failed experiment by the CIA to weaponize psychedelics by using them to embarrass or manipulate adversaries.

Then came the Nixon era, which abruptly shut down promising, questionable, and terrible lines of inquiry.

With LSD and psilocybin off the table, a small group of psychotherapists began treating patients in the late 1970s and early 1980s with MDMA. The drug was developed in 1912 by the German pharmaceutical company Merck, in the pursuit of new medications to control bleeding. Having deemed it useless for that purpose, Merck shelved the drug for decades. It was forgotten until Alexander Shulgin, an American pharmaceutical chemist, became curious about the compound. He synthesized it in his home laboratory in California and, on a lark, tried it for the first time in 1976. Marveling at the effect it had on his mind, he shared it with a psychotherapist friend.

As word spread among therapists, a few began treating patients with MDMA, but that modality did not remain legal for long. As MDMA was becoming popular as a party drug sold under a genius marketing name, ecstasy, in 1985, the DEA added it to its list of banned substances.

The following year, Rick Doblin, an American activist against drug prohibition, founded the Multidisciplinary Association for Psychedelic Studies. Doblin, who earned a doctorate in public policy from Harvard University, embarked on a decades-long quest to convince the federal government that the blanket prohibition of drugs had been deeply misguided.

MAPS's first major break came in 2001, when the Food and Drug Administration gave MAPS permission to study the efficacy of MDMA-assisted psychotherapy. That paved the way for years of expensive and complex research, much of it focused on veterans with PTSD.

In an interview, Rick told me he came to see the mental health crisis among veterans as a golden opportunity to start dismantling the war on drugs. "I like to say we don't do science, we do political science," he said. "The choice of working with veterans was very much a strategic choice about having sympathetic patients."

MAPS was also deliberate in focusing its MDMA research on PTSD. The condition is extraordinarily difficult to treat, and it's among the leading drivers of veteran disability payments, which cost taxpayers billions of dollars each year.

Toward the end of her paper, Shannon made a brief reference to MAPS's MDMA work and concluded with a forward-looking question. If shamans and medicine men had mastered the art of healing with mind-altering drugs in bygone eras, was it time for psychiatrists to rekindle those traditions?

Enthralled by the subject, Shannon emailed her paper to Dennis McKenna, an ethnopharmacologist who had collaborated extensively on psychedelics research with his brother, Terence, the author of *Food of the Gods*. (Terence McKenna died in 2000.) Shannon asked him what specialty he would recommend for a medical student wishing to work on psychedelics research.

To her delight, Dennis McKenna sent a warm response. He urged her to consider psychiatry. In her application for a residency program in psychiatry, Shannon did not disclose her interest in psychedelics. She said she was drawn to the field because it was alluring to focus on the body's least understood organ: the brain.

"Although I know much about, say, the effects of alcohol on the liver," she wrote, "I now find myself asking: 'But why does one engage in such behavior as to cause cirrhosis?'"

Shannon also emailed the psychedelics paper to Rick, the founder of MAPS. He replied teasing her for having misspelled the name of the man who developed LSD, but their correspondence evolved into a mentorship relationship and ultimately a friendship. Shannon stayed in close contact with Rick as she began a four-year residency at the VA in Loma Linda, where she specialized in addiction treatment.

During her final year of residency, Shannon gave a presentation to colleagues at the VA about MAPS's MDMA studies. MAPS clinicians were reporting something extraordinary: more than 60 percent of patients who underwent three MDMA sessions were no longer meeting the criteria for PTSD two months after the final treatment. That raised the possibility of a breakthrough for treating a condition that the VA estimates has a yearly economic burden of more than $230 billion in the United States.

The chief of psychiatry at the VA in Loma Linda was impressed.

Shannon would soon be starting a new role as an attending psychiatrist there. "We should do this here," she recalled her boss suggesting. "When you come work with us, we'll do this."

It seemed like a long shot. But in the summer of 2017, as Shannon was wrapping up her residency and preparing to start her first formal job as a psychiatrist, MAPS's MDMA study got a major boost. The Food and Drug Administration designated MDMA a breakthrough therapy for PTSD. The regulatory agency gives that label to drugs that appear to be more effective than the standard treatments, expediting the path to approve them for clinical use.

Since Shannon was an early career psychiatrist in a massive federal bureaucracy that skews conservative, getting permission to treat veterans with MDMA seemed like a pipe dream. She conferred with a colleague and close friend, Allie Kaigle, a clinical pharmacist who shared Shannon's passion for psychedelic research. Allie's interest in mental health had been shaped by her use of MDMA as a young adult. "You take this tiny little pill, and it completely changes your brain chemistry," she told me. "That was part of the reason I went into pharmacy."

Allie and Shannon learned that VA clinicians had previously proposed MDMA studies. But none had gotten past the first obstacle: getting approval from an institutional review board, a panel of experts that signs off on the soundness and safety of a medical trial.

But now that the FDA had given MDMA a tentative nod, perhaps it was time to give it another shot, they figured. Over more than a year, they huddled after hours and on weekends to draft a study proposal that would need to clear many hurdles. They would need permission from the institutional review board, the FDA, California's research advisory panel, and the DEA. Assuming that all worked out, they'd need to find veterans willing to join them in a major leap of faith.

⋙ Chris has read that adults seldom remember things that happened before the age of four or five. But he told me that his earliest memory dates back to a brutal scene when he was around eighteen months old. His enraged stepfather, who was often drunk, was beating him and his mother with a tire iron.

"It woke me to consciousness, if you will," Chris told me. By the time he was four years old, his mother, who also struggled with addiction, surrendered custody of Chris to an aunt and uncle. They were loving, doting guardians, "fantastic parents to me," Chris said. But he grew up feeling scarred by the abuse and neglect he experienced early in life, and resentful for having been separated from his siblings. "I was an angry kid," he said. "I felt kind of alone."

Loneliness led him to start drinking and smoking marijuana as a teenager, when he lacked motivation and felt rudderless, he said. But the attacks of September 11, 2001, which happened shortly before his sixteenth birthday, instilled in him a sense of purpose. He decided he would join the army or the Marine Corps the day he became eligible.

Days after his eighteenth birthday, the army offered Chris a $5,000 signing bonus and a job as an M1 Abrams tank crewman. He reported for basic training on July 3, 2003, and instantly loved the camaraderie and structure the military provided.

The day before Thanksgiving, Chris deployed to Baghdad. His base was the target of near-daily mortar attacks. Violence intensified during the final weeks of the deployment. At that moment, Chris told me, those battles did not register as particularly traumatic.

When his unit returned to the United States, Chris and his men sat through a briefing about how to readjust to life back home. He found the guidance laughable. "If you're married, don't beat your wife," he remembers a commander saying. "And if you're single, respect your parents."

Duly advised, Chris soon paid a visit to his biological mother, who was living in New Mexico at the time. She opened a bottle of liquor to welcome her nineteen-year-old son back from war. That encounter kicked off several weeks of poor choices that brought his army career to an ignominious end: when Chris reported back to his base following two weeks of postdeployment leave, a drug test showed he had done cocaine, he said. The army discharged him, setting in motion a two-year "downward spiral" during which Chris became addicted to cocaine, methamphetamine, and alcohol.

At twenty-one, in an effort to gain control of his life, Chris moved to Phoenix to live with one of his brothers. There, he fell in love with a woman. Things between them soured a month into the relationship. She was pregnant and wanted to give the baby up for adoption; Chris objected and offered to raise the baby. By the time his daughter was born in 2007, their relationship was so acrimonious that Chris was escorted out of the hospital by police officers.

"At that point, I broke," he said. "I went heavily into drugs, heavily into alcohol."

By 2016, Chris willed himself to quit meth. That made his craving for alcohol soar. "I was drinking between sixty and seventy shots a day for four years," he told me. "If I didn't drink every three to four hours, I would be violently ill."

During his years of binge drinking, Chris held down a job as a landscaper and largely kept to himself. He was drunk all the time and reeked of alcohol. Looking back, that stage of his life feels like a slow-motion suicide, a descent into an ever darker and lonelier existence with no apparent off-ramp. But a glimmer of hope appeared in the fall of 2019 in the form of an emaciated kitten that showed up at his door one night. Chris took him in, fed him, and nursed him to health. He called the cat Ghost, perhaps because that's how he had come to see himself at that point. "Through him, I was able to see that I wasn't completely devoid of life, compassion, and love," Chris told me. "I may have saved his life, but in a lot of ways, he saved mine."

To Chris's surprise, he also discovered that despite the circumstances under which he left the army, he remained eligible for health care at the VA. Doctors at the hospital in Loma Linda had warned him that he was on the brink of developing cirrhosis, a form of irreversible liver damage. Watching Ghost spring back to health spurred Chris to sign up for an inpatient rehab program. Withdrawal was excruciating. Chris spent several days hallucinating as doctors monitored his blood pressure, which rose to as high as 220 over 190.

Once he was sober, Chris still felt adrift. He befriended several of the veterans in his detox program and learned that most of them had been diagnosed with PTSD. He had long resisted that label. "To actually admit that there might be some psychological problem is to give it power over you," he said.

But Chris took a PTSD diagnostic test and scored 100 percent. It helped explain the recurring nightmares, the chronic insomnia, the inability to focus and to connect with people. The VA offered a broad range of treatments that helped him—some.

The most beneficial was a meditation course that helped steady his thoughts. But Chris was still feeling socially isolated and directionless when the VA clinicians told him about the MDMA study. He thought about it for days and scoured the internet for information. The government clinicians he had come to trust made it clear that this was an experimental protocol. He shouldn't expect that a few sessions of MDMA would be a silver bullet, they told him. There were potential downsides and a lot of unanswered questions. "They made it clear that this was an experiment," he said. "And I was going to—this is my own words—be a guinea pig."

〜〜 It took more than two years, but Shannon and Allie managed to clear all the regulatory hurdles to get their MDMA study approved. It was a tiny clinical study with no more than ten patients that borrowed heavily from the protocol MAPS had developed. The biggest contribution of the study would be to show whether MDMA therapy could be provided safely and effectively within the Veterans Affairs health care system, a vast bureaucracy that has spent billions treating PTSD.

Once all the paperwork was sorted and they identified the first handful of patients interested in participating in the study, the young VA clinicians turned their attention to a novel challenge: how to turn a government hospital room into a facility fit for a psychedelic trip.

"It was important to us to create a space that didn't feel like a sterile hospital environment," Allie said. "We didn't want this to be just another day at the VA."

The pair bought several white canvases and acrylic paint to make DIY abstract art at home. They curated special playlists and created a special ritual for each patient to start the sessions based on what they knew about them. Chris opted to sit in meditation with the clinicians for a few minutes.

The therapists set clear ground rules about what kind of touch might occur during a session. Patients could grant permission to have a hand held and to allow the therapists to rest a palm on their shoulder as a comforting gesture—or they could opt out of touch entirely. The MDMA tablets had been stored at the hospital's pharmacy in a regular pillbox. But before offering an MDMA tablet to the participants, the therapists placed it in a wooden bowl.

"It took away the sense that this was a hospital and turned it into more of a ritual," Chris said. "That really put me at ease."

After swallowing the brown pill, Chris lay down on a hospital bed outfitted with fluffy cushions and waited with a mix of exhilaration and dread for the effects to kick in. The therapists sat in silence.

Within an hour, Chris said, his powers of perception appeared to multiply, an experience that was at once awe-inspiring and overwhelming. "Everything was wide open," he said. "It kind of was like a book was flung open: here you go." The chapters of his messy past were on display, and he was able to examine each one without the sting of self-judgment and second-guessing that made taking stock of the past so painful. "I was able to just look at myself and my life through unfiltered eyes," he said. Memories were suddenly reduced to their essence, making clear to him how emotions had clouded and distorted the way he had registered formative events. "I put more emotions to certain memories the longer they had festered," he said. "A bad memory just turned into a worse one, and then it was just a terrible one."

As scenes of combat in Iraq flashed before his eyes, he was struck by how excited being a combatant had once made him feel. He simply registered that fact. Chris then replayed the sequence of events that brought his military career to an end. Then he contemplated how gutting it had felt to be cut out of his daughter's life. What came next suddenly seemed entirely reasonable—inevitable, even: the addiction, the retreat from others, the spiral of self-destructive behavior. "It was almost like seeing it from a third-person point of view and being able to just accept it," Chris said. That's not to say the memories were devoid of emotion. At times, sadness swelled within him like a rising tide. "There was a lot of crying that first day," Chris recalled. "It puts you in a vulnerable state, crying in front of other people, especially when you're kind of trained not to show that kind of emotion."

The two therapists in the room said little during the eight-hour session. Chris spent that night in the hospital. The following morning, the clinicians were back for a psychotherapy session that lasted roughly three hours. The effects of the MDMA had faded, but when Chris began to speak, he realized the instinctive inhibition and restraint that limited what he would ordinarily share with a therapist were gone. "The walls were down," he said. "I was able to talk truth and not half-truths or innuendos; I had no problem expressing emotion."

Chris cried a lot during that session. He also laughed plenty. It felt as though a glut of feelings that had been repressed for years had suddenly become unclogged.

The second MDMA session was held a little over two weeks later, just after the Christmas holiday. Chris called it his "wrecking ball day," because it demolished what remained of his emotional armor. Processing a torrent of memories that day, he was struck by how many of the events that were coming to mind made him smile. Along with the painful and distressing memories, Chris realized he had tucked away plenty of fond ones.

"There were a lot of good memories that I had repressed as well because I didn't want to deal with anything from my past," he said.

Chris relished this newfound ability to allow random memories to bubble up to the surface without becoming overwhelmed. It dawned on him that what he needed most, what would bring him closest to healing and absolution, was forgiveness. He thought about the people who had hurt him and found that forgiving them was within reach. Chris contemplated all the ways he had let himself down over the years, the damage he had done to his body, and for perhaps the first time ever, showed himself mercy. For a few days, it felt as though forgiveness was rippling through his body, coursing through his veins. It had been so hard to get to this point. But the remedy seemed stupidly obvious, and he had found it.

A few days before his third and final MDMA session, Chris watched a video on YouTube of a woman talking about acceptance. After it ended, Chris felt his body throb, and he dropped to his knees. He described feeling that a mysterious force swooped in from behind and untethered him from weights that had been holding him down his entire life.

"It was the most powerful experience of my life," Chris said. "I felt all this weight being cut off my back simultaneously." Tears streamed down his cheeks. To this day, he doesn't know whether to call that a spiritual awakening, a miracle, or a mysterious drug-induced phenomenon. But it led him to walk into the third and final MDMA session feeling serene and open to whatever it would bring. After popping the pill that day, Chris sank into an ocean of pure love.

"There was no anger toward anybody. There was no anger toward myself," he said. "There was only forgiveness and love."

∿ A few days after the third session, Chris quit his job as a land-scaper at a casino and enrolled in a community college, where he took English composition, critical thinking, and philosophy classes. "I was like a sponge," Chris said. "My mind was free for the first time from everything else, and I just soaked up all this knowledge."

Before the MDMA therapy, Chris had lacked the vision or where-withal to contemplate anything beyond getting through each day. Now he had the will and motivation to make ambitious long-term plans. The community college classes were the first step toward earning a degree in psychology. It was a field in which the years he spent in a dark place would be an asset.

"All my life experiences will allow me to understand what a patient is going through without judgment," Chris said. "I can understand the fear of opening up to somebody."

A year after the end of his MDMA sessions, Chris returned to the VA for an assessment. Clinicians said he no longer met the diagnostic criteria for PTSD, he told me. That's not to say all his problems evaporated.

When we met in the spring of 2023, Chris told me he still has debilitating nightmares, although they now happen a few times a week, no longer an everyday torment. He said he remained conflicted over whether he should try to reconnect with his daughter—and if so, when and how. He had last seen her when she was nine. She had just turned sixteen. Chris told me he desperately wanted her to know how deeply he regretted having been an absent parent. He had apologized in countless letters he wrote to her over the years—pages upon pages distilling perhaps his deepest wound—but he'd never put them in the mail.

He mentioned he had begun communicating with a woman who lives in the Midwest whom he met on a gaming app. They had been chatting for a few months, and for the first time in a long time, Chris found himself seriously contemplating dating. Whether or not things got serious, something big had shifted within him, he told me. It had been a long time since being open to the possibility of falling in love, and feeling worthy of love, had seemed possible. Now, he was starting to look at psychology programs near her hometown.

Toward the end of an hours-long conversation outside his house in La Verne, a city east of Los Angeles, I asked Chris how much weight he puts on the MDMA treatment when he looks back at how much his life changed in the months that followed. He sat silently for a while pondering my question. Then he provided what he called a conservative estimate: 80 percent. "I don't think I would have changed had it not been for the MDMA," he said, once again referring to it as a "wrecking ball" intervention. "It completely demolished the foundation of my preconceived notions of how I should operate in the world, and it allowed me to start to rebuild, but rebuild properly."

EPILOGUE

Contemplating a Magic Pill

DURING THE FINAL WEEKS OF researching this book, I traveled to the University of North Carolina at Chapel Hill to meet Dr. Bryan Roth, a prominent pharmacologist and psychiatrist who has been consumed by a fascinating mission to end depression as we know it.

Bryan began studying psychedelics decades ago, but he didn't gravitate toward compounds like LSD because he suspected that they could be administered therapeutically. He was intrigued by the way psychedelics disrupt brain activity, particularly a brain receptor that plays a key role in regulating mood and impulse control. Psychedelics, he theorized, might reveal important aspects of the body's least understood and arguably most consequential organ.

"I thought they would be a window into the brain, into consciousness," Bryan explained. "If we ultimately understood how psychedelics work, we would understand this hard problem of consciousness, of awareness, of perception."

Bryan was among the first scientists who discovered that psychedelics enhance neuroplasticity, making the interconnectedness of neural links richer. That phenomenon is now widely assumed to be at the heart of why psychedelic trips can have immediate and long-lasting therapeutic effects.

But Bryan is not part of the increasingly crowded field of researchers studying how psychedelics can be administered medicinally. In recent years, he has been consumed by a far more ambitious pursuit: determining whether the mind-bending trips psychedelics induce are an indispensable element of their healing properties.

In 2020, the Pentagon awarded Bryan's lab nearly $27 million to try to answer that question by developing new compounds that alter brain function much like psilocybin, without the perceptual side effects.

The four-year research project was funded by the Defense Advanced Research Projects Agency, a division of the Department of Defense that makes bets on high-risk, high-reward research projects. Many of the ventures DARPA has bankrolled over the years have failed. Among its most famous clunkers was a quest during the Cold War to establish a team of telepathic spies.

But the agency has played a leading role in revolutionary breakthroughs that changed the world, including the internet, GPS systems, and mRNA vaccines for COVID-19.

Dr. Matthew Pava, the DARPA official who oversees the division funding the research, told me that creating a new generation of antidepressants that kick in quickly and have long-lasting effects would be a game changer for the armed forces. In recent years, he said, 28 percent of service members medically evacuated from frontline positions are sent home after being diagnosed with a mental health condition. According to a 2021 study, roughly 23 percent of active-duty service members had been diagnosed with depressive disorder, a rate far higher than that of the civilian population.

"Treating those issues takes a while," Matthew said in an interview. "It's not like an antibiotic you can take, and go through your seven-day, fourteen-day course, and you recover."

Matthew told me he found the emerging medical literature about psychedelics enormously promising. But psychedelics are not a practical solution for the mental health crisis among veterans. For starters, he said, the protocols developed in clinical trials for MDMA- and psilocybin-assisted therapy require extensive psychotherapy, which makes them labor-intensive and costly. "Obviously, there's a major problem if you were to try to administer psychedelics to a war fighter in a frontline position. That's just not going to work."

⌁ As Bryan showed me around his thirty-person lab, which straddles two floors of a modern redbrick building on the university's medical school campus, I referred to his DARPA-funded research as a moon shot. He corrected me. "We call it a *Mars shot*," Bryan said, chuckling. "Because we've been to the moon."

The first step of the Mars shot entailed using powerful computers to create millions of hypothetical new psychedelic compounds that, like psilocybin, would be expected to bind to a receptor in the brain known as 5-HT2A. Using sophisticated predictive modeling techniques, Bryan's team then winnowed down that massive catalog of new compounds to several hundred finalists that showed the most promise. Among them, dozens emerged as finalists that made it to the decisive step: the stoned mice test.

The scientists administered the drugs to rodents in an effort to determine which ones appear to alter perception and behavior in hopes of finding a few that don't. How can you tell whether a mouse gets high? The first thing scientists look for is head twitching, Bryan explained. Tripping mice explore the holes in their cage with curiosity, often sticking their noses in them. Some also move in a way reminiscent of moonwalking. When a new drug induces some or all of those effects, the lab concludes it has created a brand-new psychedelic— paid for by the federal government. Those get discarded as failures and never make it out of the lab. The researchers then move on to the next compound, hoping it will induce no noticeable change in the behavior of their mice.

If he manages to create such a compound, and it is deemed safe and promising enough to test on people, Bryan intends to team up with a pharmaceutical company to conduct human trials. That stage of the research would cost millions and last several years. Call it a moon shot or a Mars shot. If the quest to create a psilocybin-mimicking antidepressant succeeds, it may well take the wind out of the sails of the psychedelic renaissance and undermine those working to end the war on drugs.

〰 When I first spoke to Bryan a few months before our meeting, I asked him whether he had personal experience with psychedelics. He told me it was a topic he doesn't discuss publicly. Sitting across his desk, I wondered whether he would be similarly guarded when I asked how mental illness has shaped his life. He was not.

"My mother had schizophrenia," Bryan told me. She went unmedicated for years because the side effects of antipsychotic drugs were noxious. His mother's delusions made for a very chaotic childhood. When he and his siblings sensed a violent outburst coming, they hid the kitchen knives. The day President Kennedy was assassinated, she grew paranoid. Believing that the family would be targeted next, she bundled the kids into the car and drove to a nearby city.

Bryan's sister battled addiction and depression much of her life. She died by suicide after taking an overdose of her antidepressants. While he has not experienced crippling depression, Bryan said that for many years he struggled to make sense of "a lot of noise in my head." The best antidote he found to tame an overactive mind that made it hard to focus was Zen meditation, which he practices daily for as long as three or four hours.

His wife, he shared, has lived with severe depression most of her life. Antidepressants have been helpful, but she continues to suffer enormously. Witnessing the suffering of loved ones drove his interest in branches of medicine that study human behavior and the pharmacological interventions that shape it.

"It would be wonderful for me if we invented ourselves out of a profession," he said. "To actually cure depression—who would possibly be against that?"

It's hard to argue with the notion that easing human suffering on a massive scale is a worthwhile goal that could save countless lives and unlock vast human potential. But for reasons I couldn't pinpoint in the moment, the question unsettled me. There was something unseemly about the federal government, which spent decades demonizing psychedelics, suddenly backing research that seeks to copy part of their code in order to create a lab-produced sanitized analogue. If Pentagon-funded research one day makes treating depression and PTSD as easy as taking a course of antibiotics to stamp out a bacterial infection, what would that do to our collective moral compass? Might it make it chillingly easy to commit—or bear witness to—atrocities and then walk away unscathed? Could it tempt us to take it a step further one day by enabling people to opt out of the grieving process when a loved one passes?

Shouldn't overcoming trauma require letting pain and distress run its course? If we become much better at metabolizing suffering, would we harm others more wantonly? Awful memories often set the trajectory of extraordinary lives. I asked Bryan if he had entertained some of these moral questions as part of his research. After a long pause, he told me he found it doubtful that we're close to designing a silver bullet psychiatric drug.

As things stand, he said, the causes and nature of depression remain poorly understood. At best, his work may make a dent in human misery. "The goal of the physician is to relieve human suffering," he said. "That's our focus."

〰〰 For weeks after our conversation, my mind kept returning to the idea of a magic pill capable of vanquishing depression and other maladies of the mind in a flash.

It was tempting to contemplate how many lives such a drug could save. I asked several friends who have experienced suicidal ideation whether they would have taken the pill Bryan hopes to create, had it been available on their darkest day. Most conveyed a version of what I felt. In the depths of despair, an instant off-ramp would likely have been irresistible. But in retrospect, they said they deeply appreciate the ways in which suffering has shaped their values and temperament. Like me, they have come to see depression as a misfortune that can be a powerful teacher, a curse that often offers blessings.

It took years to reach that conclusion. Looking back, it's evident the early seeds were planted the night Silvia handed me that first cup of ayahuasca in Brazil. The journey that began that night has been far from easy. But it has left me with deep reverence for the mysterious compounds we call psychedelics. In the wrong hands, they can be as dangerous as a drunk surgeon with a trembling hand. And, unfortunately, there is no shortage of shoddy practitioners, people who are in over their heads or downright reckless.

But when administered by a steady, wise guide, in a safe setting, I have seen psychedelics transform lives—including my own. With proper safeguards, psychoactive compounds have the potential to reduce suffering on a large scale.

Whether that potential is seized remains to be seen. While the movement to decriminalize psychedelics has made enormous headway in recent years, the web of laws and programs and beliefs that make up the war on drugs remains firmly entrenched. The likely approval by the FDA of MDMA and psilocybin as medicine ought to be a catalyst for a frank and evidence-based conversation about the risks and benefits of all drugs. Such a reckoning would benefit from greater candor about our personal use of these substances. This would help dial down the hype while giving people who are suffering significant hope.

What they have done within me will always be, to some extent, mysterious and ineffable. Yet there's much I have been able to put into words. Psychedelics gave me a granular understanding of the anatomy of my depression. Depression, at its core, is a disease of tormenting thoughts that become the building blocks of our belief system. When deluded beliefs shape our choices, we inevitably create fresh sources of suffering. Understanding this dynamic does not provide an instant reprieve. But it does offer a road map out of darkness. We discover the mind is more malleable than seemed apparent. We realize we are not condemned to be lifelong hostages of a poisoned well of thoughts.

Had it not been for psychedelics, I'm doubtful I would have found value in a spiritual practice. After my first retreat, I began meditating daily. That ancient practice made me a better student of my mind and has allowed me to move a bit more gently through a turbulent world. The glimpse of divinity some of these ceremonies provided made me a believer in prayer. I turn to prayer often these days, finding more solace than answers, a certain peace if not quite miracles.

But perhaps most significantly, psychedelics showed me that my depression, at its peak, was a clarion call of unmet needs. Chief among them was a dearth of love, an inability to connect intimately with someone who could be a safe harbor, a solitude deepened by a mix of cynicism, fear, and a sense of unworthiness.

On a crisp spring morning in San Francisco, I set out to override those by making a grand gesture I had been secretly planning for months. I had flown out with Steve for a long weekend, having falsely told him the purpose of the trip was to attend a conference. The morning after we flew in, we went our separate ways and made plans to meet in the afternoon.

I walked a few miles from downtown, where we stayed, to the Golden Gate Bridge. I had thought about the bridge often in the preceding months, spurred by the dreamlike vision I had during the queer retreat in Peru. I felt called to retrace those footsteps in real life, to ponder the path of the more than 1,700 people who had put an end to their misery by plunging five hundred feet into the icy water that flows under the landmark.

The early hours of the day in April 2023 had been cloudless, but a misty fog blanketed the bridge when I started walking along the pedestrian path toward its midpoint. I passed by several blue signs appealing to the despondent. "THE CONSEQUENCES OF JUMPING

FROM THIS BRIDGE ARE FATAL AND TRAGIC," one read, providing a number to text in order to reach a crisis counselor. I observed a stainless steel mesh net that stretches out 20 feet along the bridge's 1.7-mile length, part of a $400 million initiative designed to make jumping from the iconic suicide destination harder. Reaching the center, I rested my arms on the railing and stared into the fog, so thick now it had rendered invisible the bay I had just seen brimming with life on an unseasonably warm day.

Observing the newly installed mesh, I took stock of the safety net I had managed to build for myself over the past five years. I said a silent prayer and walked back toward the bay with about an hour to spare before meeting Steve at Baker Beach.

I'd told him we would be meeting a friend for a picnic there. But that was a ruse. Shortly after Steve found me sitting on the beach, which has a splendid view of the bridge, a group of female mariachis dressed in royal blue began walking toward us. Soon after falling for him two years earlier, I had begun to fantasize how I might one day propose. I imagined doing it with uncharacteristic flair, to compensate for the years I spent feeling ashamed of being drawn to men. When the idea of hiring mariachis first crossed my mind, I dismissed it as outlandishly corny. But weeks earlier, as my plans were taking shape, I called a couple of mariachi bands in the Bay Area and instantly connected with Lilia Chávez, the founder of an all-female troupe called Mariachi Femenil. I asked her if they played "Si Nos Dejan," the song that had become Steve's favorite on the playlist I made the week we met. It was in their repertoire. And they were available the day we would be in town.

When the blare of the trumpets grew closer and the seven musicians stopped a few feet from us, Steve looked confused. The scene was so surreal and unexpected, he didn't immediately identify the song. It only made sense once I fished a ring box from my tote bag, dropped to one knee, and asked him to marry me. He leaped over to kiss me, looking moved and mortified in equal measure.

I had heard that song countless times. But as Steve accepted the gold band, my heart stirred as I found new layers of meaning in the lyrics of a beloved anthem of defiant joy.

If they let us, we can move to a new world, where you and I may yet find happiness. If they let us, we'll find a corner near the heavens . . . If they let us, we'll turn clouds into velvet . . .

A NOTE OF GRATITUDE

WRITING THIS BOOK WAS ENORMOUSLY hard. It was also a deeply rewarding and cathartic process made possible by a long list of people who saw value in what I was trying to do. They kept me afloat with gestures of faith, solidarity, generosity, and wisdom. This is a partial accounting of my gratitude and their role in bringing this book to life. I thank the universe for making Silvia Polivoy my maiden guide to the wondrous world of ayahuasca. Her warmth and conviction helped put an end to my darkest night. When I set out to learn more about the lives of two of my late grandparents, I reached out to a few relatives tentatively. Eduardo Martínez, Himelda Martínez, and Hernando Londoño graciously shared their memories of a difficult family history, allowing me to leave a record of two extraordinary elders. Yawakashau Yawanawá and his extraordinarily talented and joyous family deepened my sense of wonder and reverence for the Amazon rainforest. The many songs I recorded during my trip to Mushu Inu village have become my antidepressant of choice. Ayahuasca retreats can be extraordinary incubators of deep, nourishing friendships. The greatest gift of my would-be Buddhist ayahuasca retreat in Peru was befriending Sonia Kreitzer and Tashima Wildrose, two giant-hearted women I hope to call close friends for many years to come. Públio Valle, who led the first queer retreat at the Temple of the Way of Light, has been a steadying force during moments of turbulence and often soothed my soul by breaking into song. Dr. Shannon Remick trusted me to tell a fascinating and sensitive chapter of this history, as did Chris Conlogue, who one day will make a fine and empathetic therapist. I have deep gratitude and admiration for both. At the *New York Times*, Caroline Que was the initial champion and enabler of this project. Juliana Barbassa did the lion's share of the editing early on, sharpening my ideas and prose with an exacting eye and a clear sense of what this book could and should be. Her role was invaluable—and it made our friendship ever more so. Nancy Lee boosted me with the strength and common sense she radiates. Lis Moriconi helped me navigate some trying years in Brazil with tenderness and wisdom, which were on display when she provided early feedback on the manuscript. Julie Tate fact-checked and gut-checked the book with her trademark precision and incisiveness. My colleagues Mitch Smith and Liriel Higa and Ellen Barry were among the first readers of *Trippy* and each provided valuable feedback and suggestions. Dr. Joshua S. Siegel at Washington University in St. Louis generously offered to read the manuscript to help me be precise about medical and scientific issues. Todd Shuster, my agent, has been a wise sounding board and advocate. I have forgiven him for failing to warn me just how hard it is to write a damn book. Ryan Doherty at Celadon took a gamble on a first-time author and has been unfailingly supportive, patient, and sharp as an editor. I was lucky to be in the first cohort of the Ferriss—UC Berkeley Psychedelic Journalism Fellowship, which helped fund my reporting and provided valuable guidance. I realize it's a bit strange to add a dog who will never read this to the acknowledgments. But Hugo was a steadfast companion during long hours spent banging away at the keyboard, oftentimes writing myself into a blur of tears. There aren't enough treats for such a good dog. Last but certainly not least, I am indebted to my husband, Steven Friedenberg, who had no idea the wild journey he was signing up for after agreeing to go on a bike-ride date on a weekend that altered the course of our lives. I'm not always easy to love, I know. But I am so tremendously lucky to have found you, to have impulsively said "I love you" a week in, and to be spending this one and precious life by your side.

AUTHOR'S NOTE

I GREW UP IN THE shadow of the war on drugs. The 1980s and 1990s were scary and volatile decades in Colombia, where I was born and raised. The cocaine trade was at the heart of a messy armed conflict that killed thousands, displaced millions, and traumatized virtually every Colombian of my generation.

The darkness of that era made me steer clear of drugs, which I long regarded as a scourge. I saw no redeeming qualities in these substances that had been outlawed long before I was born. Drug dealers and users, in my view, were contempt-worthy people with blood on their hands.

Had the war on drugs been won early in my adult life, I might have regarded that as a blessing. But the journey I chronicle in this book forced me to reconsider much of what I learned about drugs as a child.

For starters, it was humbling to learn how Indigenous people have used and understood psychoactive plants for centuries. To them, these mysterious compounds are sacred tools that keep them connected to their ancestors and to spirit realms. They find it absurd that governments across the world saw fit to outlaw plant-based compounds and treat them on par with dangerous and addictive drugs like heroin.

As I began spending time with spiritual communities that have appropriated and reimagined the ritualistic use of psychedelics, I was skeptical. At first glance, many members of these communities came across as nutty, untethered from reality, and even a bit cultish. But sitting in on their rituals, sometimes as a participant and sometimes as an observer, I gained an appreciation for the value of a spiritual practice. This forced me to think long and hard about my complicated history with Catholicism, organized religion, and faith. I began dabbling in prayer during these ceremonies, tentatively at first. But I soon discovered that prayer could bring enormous solace, particularly to a mind prone to depression.

It is no small irony that I lost any appetite for alcohol overnight after my first ayahuasca retreat. It took an altered state with a substance the United States classifies as a drug more dangerous than cocaine to understand, rationally and viscerally, how harmful drinking was for my physical and mental health.

This book is being published at a time when laws and attitudes about drug use are shifting rapidly in the United States and much of the world. As of early 2024, more than half of Americans were living in states where marijuana was legal. Cannabis, consumed medicinally and recreationally, has become a big business.

Psychedelics—once among the most stigmatized class of drugs— have turned a growing number of skeptics into enthusiasts. Among leading psychiatrists, there is little doubt that psychedelics stand to play a major role in easing our mental health care crisis. By legalizing psychedelics, Oregon and Colorado recently made a significant dent in prohibition and will soon give us a sense of the pitfalls and opportunities that might come with broader legalization.

None of this means that the war on drugs is in its final days. Drugs continue to kill, harm, and sow mayhem in Colombia and around the globe. Governments continue to spend billions fighting addiction and drug trafficking. There are no easy policy solutions that would bring it to a neat and speedy end.

But there is an opportunity to rethink the rules and frontlines of this battle.

As you put down this book, I hope you will join me in reconsidering the role drugs have played in your life. Speaking more candidly about this difficult subject may challenge longtime assumptions and lead to a more pragmatic approach. I am under no illusion that the war on drugs will be over in my lifetime. But it is my heartfelt prayer that this book contributes to greater discernment between the drugs that harm and those that heal.

NOTES

Preface

1 **Robert Fitzgerald walked into:** Robert Fitzgerald, interview with the author, October 26, 2022.

3 **"These medicines shouldn't be restricted":** Whitney Lasseter, interview with the author, October 28, 2022.

3 **In 2021, at least 48,183 people killed themselves:** Deborah M. Stone, "Notes from the Field: Recent Changes in Suicide," *Morbidity and Mortality Weekly Report* 72, no. 6 (February 10, 2023): 160–2, https://www.cdc.gov/mmwr /volumes/72/wr/mm7206a4.htm.

3 **To put it into perspective, that figure is:** Vincent Milano, "FBI Releases 2021 Crime Statistics," Homeland Security Digital Library, October 5, 2022, https://www.hsdl.org/c/fbi-releases-2021-crime-statistics/#:~:text=The%20 number%20of%20murders%20increased,the%2029.4%25%20increase%20 in%202020.

4 **Twenty-four percent of Americans described:** Megan Brenan, "Americans' Reported Mental Health at New Low; More Seek Help," Gallup, January 24, 2023, https://news.gallup.com/poll/467303/americans-reported-mental -health-new-low-seek-help.aspx.

4 **A broad majority of Americans report feeling deeply frustrated:** Mallory Newall, "Americans Are Unhappy with the Country's Mental Health Care System," Ipsos, June 16, 2022, https://www.ipsos.com/en-us/news-polls /americans-unhappy-mental-health-united-states-061622.

4 **The journalist Michael Pollan turbocharged:** Michael Pollan, *How to Change Your Mind: What the New Science of Psychedelics Teaches Us About Consciousness, Dying, Addiction, Depression, and Transcendence* (New York: Penguin, 2019).

4 **Regulators at the Food and Drug Administration:** Rick Doblin, MAPS Bulletin, Winter 2017, https://maps.org/news/bulletin/from-the-desk-of-rick -doblin-ph-d-winter-2017.

4 **and psilocybin, the psychoactive compound in psychedelic mushrooms:** Tracy Chung, "Compass Pathways Receives FDA Breakthrough Therapy Designation for Psilocybin Therapy for Treatment-Resistant Depression," Compass Pathways, October 23, 2018, https://compasspathways.com/compass -pathways-receives-fda-breakthrough-therapy-designation-for-psilocybin -therapy-for-treatment-resistant-depression.

4 **The Department of Veterans Affairs has begun administering psychedelics:** Ernesto Londoño, "After Six-Decade Hiatus, Experimental Psychedelic Therapy Returns to the V.A.," *New York Times*, June 24, 2022, https://www .nytimes.com/2022/06/24/us/politics/psychedelic-therapy-veterans.html.

4 **The federal government in 2021 began to fund research:** NIH Catalyst Staff, "Psychedelic Medicine Returns to the NIH," NIH Intramural Research Program, March 16, 2023, https://irp.nih.gov/catalyst/31/2/the-sig-beat -psychedelic-medicine.

5 **Dr. Joshua Gordon, the director of the National Institute of Mental Health:** Joshua Gordon, interview with the author, February 16, 2023.

5 **Since 2019, venture capitalists have provided:** Andrew Jacobs, "With Promise of Legalization, Psychedelic Companies Joust over Future Profits," *New York Times*, October 25, 2022, https://www.nytimes.com/2022/10/25/health /psychedelic-drug-therapy-patents.html.

5 **One of the most expensive ones, which promises:** "Rythmia Scholarship," Rythmia, https://www.rythmia.com/scholarship.html.

6 **Voters in Oregon in 2020 approved:** "Oregon Measure 109 Election Results: Legalize Psilocybin," *New York Times*, December 4, 2020, https://www

.nytimes.com/interactive/2020/11/03/us/elections/results-oregon-measure-109
-legalize-psilocybin.html.

6 **Between 2017 and 2022, lawmakers have introduced:** Joshua Siegel, James
E. Daily, Demetrius A. Perry, and Ginger E. Nicol, "Psychedelic Drug Legislative
Reform and Legalization in the US," *JAMA Psychiatry* 80, no. 1 (2023): 77–83,
https://jamanetwork.com/journals/jamapsychiatry/article-abstract/2799268.

1: A Twisted Ritual

19 **The promising field had flourished:** Robin Carhart-Harris, "The Therapeutic Potential of Psychedelic Drugs: Past, Present, and Future," *Neuropsycho-
pharmacology* 42, no. 11 (April 26, 2017): 2105–13, https://www.ncbi.nlm.nih
.gov/pmc/articles/PMC5603818/.

20 **The first link I clicked led to a video:** "Ayahuasca Retreat in Brazil at
Spirit Vine Center, Introduction," YouTube video, 9:40, posted by Spirit Vine
Ayahuasca Retreat Center, September 7, 2011, https://www.youtube.com/watch
?v=FG3A86c14Ds.

2: "Have a Good Journey"

23 **The first participant I met at Spirit Vine:** Quotes and descriptions
in this chapter are drawn from the author's memory and notes, February 2018.

31 **"I cannot live like that," he wrote:** Ernesto Londoño, "Returning Home,
a Veteran War Reporter Wrestled with Old Wounds," *New York Times*, December 15, 2014, https://www.nytimes.com/2014/12/16/opinion/returning-home-a
-veteran-war-reporter-wrestled-with-old-wounds.html.

37 **Recent advances in neuroimaging have given:** Hilary P. Blumberg, "Brain
Scans as Predictors of Suicide," Yale Medicine, Spring 2017, https://medicine.yale
.edu/news/yale-medicine-magazine/article/brain-scans-as-predictors-of-suicide/.

37 **"Brain activity becomes less predictable, faster":** Robin Carhart-
Harris, interview with the author, November 5, 2022.

38 **the term *psychedelic*, which was coined in the 1950s:** Douglas Martin,
"Humphry Osmond, 86, Who Sought Medicinal Value in Psychedelic Drugs,
Dies," *New York Times*, February 22, 2004, https://www.nytimes.com/2004
/02/22/us/humphry-osmond-86-who-sought-medicinal-value-in-psychedelic
-drugs-dies.html.

38 **But the nascent field soon fell into disrepute:** Don Lattin, *The Harvard Psychedelic Club: How Timothy Leary, Ram Dass, Huston Smith, and Andrew Weil Killed the Fifties and Ushered in a New Age for America* (New York: HarperCollins, 2011).

38 **As more young people took psychedelics:** Abigail M. Stanger, "'Moral Panic' in the Sixties: The Rise and Rapid Declination of LSD in American Society," *Cardinal Edge* 1, no. 2 (2021), https://ir.library.louisville.edu/cgi/viewcontent .cgi?article=1072&context=tce#:~:text=Although%20LSD%20became%20 revered%20as,measures%20which%20ultimately%20declared%20no.

39 **"Psychedelics, used responsibly and with proper caution":** Stanislav Grof, *LSD Psychotherapy* (San Jose, CA: Multidisciplinary Association for Psychedelic Studies, 2008).

3: A Lineage of Unstable Minds

44 **"We're at a really exciting time in the field of psychiatric genetics":** Erin C. Dunn, interview with the author, August 25, 2022.

45 **They have documented this by studying the descendants:** Rachel Yehuda, "Intergenerational Transmission of Trauma Effects: Putative Role of Epigenetic Mechanisms," *World Psychiatry* 17, no. 3 (October 2018): 243–57, https://www.ncbi.nlm.nih.gov/pmc/articles/PMC6127768/.

46 **He had an extraordinary talent for math:** Eduardo Martínez, interview with the author, March 31, 2022.

50 **Dr. Uribe pulled a thick book titled:** Morris Fishbein, *Family Encyclopedia of Medicine and Health* (Westport, CT: H. S. Stuttman, 1978).

51 **"My mom convinced us that *Papi* suffered enormously":** Margarita Martínez, interview with the author, June 6, 2022.

55 **"My mother realized that she didn't know":** Hernando Londoño, interview with the author, October 9, 2020.

56 **Curious to learn more about the roots:** Name withheld, interview with the author, May 30, 2022.

4: The Yawanawá

61 **Surely a responsible adult would intervene:** Descriptions and quotes from Yawanawá community members in this chapter are drawn from interviews with the author and interviews during a trip in February 2022.

66 **Ayahuasca is prepared by boiling crushed chunks:** Simon Ruffell, Nige Netzband, Catherine Bird, Allan H. Young, and Mario F. Juruena, "The Pharmacological Interaction of Compounds in Ayahuasca: A Systematic Review," *Brazilian Journal of Psychiatry* 42, no. 6 (November–December 2020): 646–56, https://www.ncbi.nlm.nih.gov/pmc/articles/PMC7678905/.

66 **Jeremy Narby, a Canadian anthropologist:** Jeremy Narby, *The Cosmic Serpent* (New York: Putnam, 2000).

67 **Esther Jean Langdon, a Tulane-trained anthropologist:** Esther Jean Langdon, interview with the author, November 19, 2021.

67 **Steve Beyer, a religious studies scholar:** Steve Beyer, "On the Origins of Ayahuasca," *Singing to the Plants* (blog), April 25, 2012, https://singingtotheplants .com/2012/04/on-origins-of-ayahuasca/.

67 **Another prominent challenger of the millennial:** Bernd Brabec de Mori, "Tracing Hallucinations: Contributing to a Critical Ethnohistory of Ayahuasca Usage in the Peruvian Amazon," ResearchGate, January 2011, https://www .researchgate.net/publication/321038305_Tracing_Hallucinations_-_Contributing _to_a_Critical_Ethnohistory_of_Ayahuasca_Usage_in_the_Peruvian_Amazon.

67 **Evgenia Fotiou, a cultural anthropologist in the United States:** Evgenia Fotiou, interview with the author, May 5, 2022.

68 **The oldest written accounts of ayahuasca ceremonies:** Jesse Hudson, "Ayahuasca and Globalization," NEIP, March 28, 2011, https://neip.info/novo/wp -content/uploads/2017/11/Hudson_J-Ayahuasaca_and_Globalization_2011.pdf.

5: Holy Ayahuasca

77 **"I don't disown everything we did, the radicalism":** Alex Polari, interview with the author, December 9, 2022.

78 **In the years following the supposed prophecy:** William Barnard, *Liquid Light: Ayahuasca Spirituality and the Santo Daime Tradition* (New York: Columbia University Press, 2022), https://cup.columbia.edu/book/liquid -light/9780231186612.

79 **The first song that came to him was titled:** Mestre Irineu, "Lua Branca," Nossa Irmandade, https://nossairmandade.com/hymn/191/LuaBranca.

82 **The group, which included government officials:** "Ata de Reunião do Conselho Federal de Entorpecentes-CONFEN," Santo Daime, August 24, 1992, https://www.santodaime.org/site-antigo/institucional/ata_confen.htm.

82 **Much of the outcry was driven by allegations:** Alicia Castilla, *Santo Daime: Fanatismo e Lavagem Cerebral* (Rio de Janeiro: Imago, 1995).

82 **In a lengthy written rebuttal at the time:** Alex Polari, letter to Secretário Nacional do CEFLURIS, January 6, 1995, https://www.mestreirineu.org /argumento_alex.htm.

83 **In 2004, the National Council on Drug Policy:** Resolução CONAD nº 5, April 11, 2004, https://www.normasbrasil.com.br/norma/resolucao-5-2004 _100836.html.

86 **One striking initiation story came from William Barnard:** William Barnard, interview with the author, September 19, 2022.

6: The Tripping Buddhist

93 **The red flags were there from the start:** Descriptions of events during the October 2021 retreat are drawn from the author's recollections and notes.

94 **Many of us had read her memoir:** Spring Washam, *A Fierce Heart: Finding Strength, Courage, and Wisdom in Any Moment* (Berkeley, CA: Parallax Press, 2017).

94 **"Ayahuasca is a powerful doctor":** "How to Raise Your Vibration with Ayahuasca," YouTube video, 14:10, posted by Lotus Vine Journeys, September 7, 2021, https://www.youtube.com/watch?v=TimFbxVz9fo.

97 **He was the protagonist of the 2016 documentary:** *The Last Shaman*, directed by Raz Degan (New York: Abramorama, 2016), 77 min.

98 **"The plants began to teach me":** Pepe Franchini Vásquez, interview with the author, October 23, 2021.

99 **It was only days later, when she and I sat down to talk:** Fame Chanel, interview with the author, October 27, 2021.

105 **Katari and Herbert Quintero had become:** Sina California (pseudonym), "TRIGGER WARNING: Sexual Assault by Shaman," Facebook video, 13:08, March 30, 2021, https://www.facebook.com/watch/?v=285061579847858.

7: A Rape in the Rainforest

111 **Michelle Sánchez met the man:** Michelle Sánchez, interview with the author, September 23, 2022.

112 **His website, featuring a photo of Victor:** "About the Founder," Kambo Jungle Expeditions, https://kambojungleexpeditions.vangolde.com/?page_id=27.

112 **Kambo was a treatment of last resort for Tabatha Marie Hammer:** Tabatha Marie Hammer, interview with the author, May 10, 2022.

113 **Kailey Horsley, a third retreat participant:** Kailey Horsley, interview with the author, May 6, 2022.

113 **Starting in 2017, he and Natasha began:** Natasha Devi, "Peace Love and Kambo," Love and Devi, http://www.loveanddevi.com/kambo-practitioners.html.

120 **Soon after arriving in the United States, she posted:** Kailey Horsley, "Trigger Warning—Sexual Assault and Rape," Facebook video, November 21, 2021, https://www.facebook.com/kailey.robinson.71/videos/572263610541980 (video removed).

121 **Daniela Peluso, an anthropologist who:** Daniela Peluso, "Ayahuasca's Attractions and Distractions: Examining Sexual Seduction in Shaman-Participant Interactions," in *Ayahuasca Shamanism in the Amazon and Beyond*, ed. Beatriz C. Labate and Clancy Cavnar (Oxford: Oxford University Press, 2014), 231–55.

122 **As it turns out, Victor had been accused of rape:** SF Weekly Staff, "S.F. State Grad Alleges Rape in Peru; Peruvian Media Circus Ensues," *SF Weekly*, February 10, 2010, https://www.sfweekly.com/archives/s-f-state-grad -alleges-rape-in-peru-peruvian-media-circus-ensues/article_b40746b8-2c6f -5fa7-a010-0ca67de760d5.html.

123 **When I got her on the phone, the maestra:** Sara Ramírez, interview with the author, October 11, 2022.

123 **Natasha told me that she and Victor:** Natasha Devi, interview with the author, October 12, 2022.

124 **"These women, honestly, completely destroyed":** Victor Escobar, interview with the author, October 12, 2022.

8: "Boot Camp Healing"

129 **The first to bring up suicidal ideation:** The account of the April 2022 retreat is drawn from the author's recollections and notes, having been a participant.

130 **The Temple opened in 2007 in a patch of thick:** Matthew Watherston, interview with the author, May 26, 2022.

134 **A 2022 mental health survey by the Trevor Project:** Amit Paley, "2022 National Survey on LGBTQ Youth Mental Health," Trevor Project, 2022, https://www.thetrevorproject.org/survey-2022.

135 **They told me suicidal people are often:** Yana Calou, interview with the author, December 15, 2022.

135 **Públio said, he has found value in meeting mentions:** Públio Valle, interview with the author, April 11, 2022.

136 **Públio's colleague Juliana Bizare told me:** Juliana Bizare, interview with the author, April 11, 2022.

136 **Holly, the nonbinary journalist, told me:** Holly Regan, interview with the author, May 26, 2022.

138 **As an adult, he said, he felt he carried a form:** Ed, interview with the author, April 13, 2022.

140 **Midway through the retreat, I sat next to Fia:** Fia Duda, interview with the author, June 23, 2022.

144 **On a sunny afternoon, I sat down with Toni:** Maestro Toni Lopez, interview with the author, April 16, 2022.

9: Chasing Miracles in Costa Rica

147 **The first two things that caught my eye:** Scenes and events in this chapter are largely drawn from the author's recollections and notes, having been a guest at Rythmia in July 2022.

151 **I was familiar with Gerry's story, having read his memoir:** Gerard Powell, *Sh*t the Moon Said: A Story of Sex, Drugs, and Ayahuasca* (Deerfield Beach, FL: Health Communications, 2018).

157 **He told me that stem cell replacement therapy has:** Paul Knoepfler, interview with the author, August 15, 2022.

162 **So I found myself asking Gerry gentler questions:** Gerard Powell, interview with the author, July 10, 2022.

165 **Dr. Allan Varela, a senior official at Costa Rica's health ministry:** Allan Varela, interview with the author, August 26, 2022.

165 **I tracked down a former Rythmia yoga teacher:** Candice Marie Fox, interview with the author, July 20, 2022.

166 **That's what happened to Jenna Williams:** Jenna Williams, interview with the author, July 24, 2022.

167 **Soon after getting in touch with Jenna, I heard from Zinlynn:** Zinlynn Somerville, interview with the author, July 21, 2022.

10: The Ayahuasca Churches

175 **Surely the driver had made a wrong turn:** Aaron Goldman, interview with the author, October 17, 2022.

176 **That morning, Jonathan and Jane:** Jonathan Goldman, interview with the author, August 1, 2022.

177 **Jane told me:** Jane Seligson, interview with the author, October 3, 2022.

177 **they sued the government:** "Supreme Court Case," Centro Espírita Beneficente União do Vegetal, https://udvusa.org/supreme-court-case.

178 **"It was a bold move," Liza Goitein:** Liza Goitein, interview with the author, February 2, 2023.

178 **In 1981, Theodore Olson, who was then:** Peyote exemption for Native American Church, Department of Justice, December 22, 1981, https://www.justice.gov/file/22846/download#:~:text=%C2%A7%201307.31%2C%20which%20provides%3A%202,peyote%20are%20exempt%20from%20registration.

178 **The Supreme Court sided with Oregon:** Employment Division v. Smith, 494 U.S. 872 (1990), Supreme Court ruling summary, National Constitution Center, https://constitutioncenter.org/the-constitution/supreme-court-case-library/employment-division-v-smith.

179 **Heeding their call, in 1993, Congress set a higher bar:** Religion Freedom and Restoration Act, November 16, 1993, https://www.congress.gov/bill/103rd-congress/house-bill/1308#:~:text=Religious%20Freedom%20Restoration%20Act%20of%201993%20%2D%20Prohibits%20any%20agency%2C%20department,government%20may%20burden%20a%20person's.

179 **President Bill Clinton hailed the law:** Peter Steinfels, "Clinton Signs Law Protecting Religious Practices," *New York Times*, November 17, 1993, https://www.nytimes.com/1993/11/17/us/clinton-signs-law-protecting-religious-practices.html.

179 **The following year, Congress passed:** American Indian Religious Freedom Act Amendments of 1994, H.R.4230, 103rd Cong. (1993–1994), https://www.congress.gov/bill/103rd-congress/house-bill/4230.

179 **In its complaint, the church stated that:** Centro Espírita Beneficente União do Vegetal v. Janet Reno, complaint, November 21, 2000.

180 **The case made it to the Supreme Court:** Linda Greenhouse, "Sect Allowed to Import Its Hallucinogenic Tea," *New York Times*, February 22,

2006, https://www.nytimes.com/2006/02/22/politics/sect-allowed-to-import-its
-hallucinogenic-tea.html.

180 **Seeking to attain the same benefit:** The Church of the Holy Light of
the Queen v. Michael Mukasey, complaint, August 12, 2008.

180 **In a twenty-two-page ruling, Judge Panner provided:** Church of
Holy Light of the Queen v. Michael B. Mukasey, et al., 615 F. Supp. 2d 1210
(D. Or. 2009), https://www.govinfo.gov/content/pkg/USCOURTS-ord-1_08-cv
-03095/pdf/USCOURTS-ord-1_08-cv-03095-1.pdf.

183 **Jonathan posits that each person is a soul that:** Jonathan Goldman,
Gift of the Body: A Multi-Dimensional Guide to Energy Anatomy, Grounded Spir-
ituality and Living Through the Heart (Ashland, OR: Essential Light Institute,
2014).

189 **In my lifetime, church membership in the United States:** Jeffrey
Jones, "U.S. Church Membership Falls Below Majority for First Time," Gallup, March 29, 2021, https://news.gallup.com/poll/341963/church-membership
-falls-below-majority-first-time.aspx.

189 **A 2019 study by the Pew Research Center found that:** Joey Marshall,
"Are Religious People Happier, Healthier? Our New Global Study Explores This
Question," Pew Research Center, January 31, 2019, https://www.pewresearch
.org/short-reads/2019/01/31/are-religious-people-happier-healthier-our-new
-global-study-explores-this-question/.

11: The New Psychedelic Churches Ministering to Veterans

193 **Whitney Lasseter was raised by a devout Southern Baptist:** Whitney
Lasseter, interview with the author, October 28, 2022.

194 **After the DEA was forced to establish a regulatory:** "Drug Enforcement
Administration Diversion Control Division Guidance Document," US Department of Justice, November 20, 2020, https://www.deadiversion.usdoj.gov/GDP/
(DEA-DC-5)(EO-DEA-007)(Version2)RFRA_Guidance_(Final)_11-20-2020
.pdf.

194 **Daniel Peterson, a lawyer in Washington, DC:** Danny Peterson, interview with the author, August 3, 2022.

195 **On its website, Soul Quest presents a forty-six-page holy text ti-**
tled: Anonymous, *Ayahuasca Manifesto: The Spirit of Ayahuasca and Its Planetary*

Mission (Orlando: Soul Quest, 2011), https://www.ayahuascachurches.org/wp -content/uploads/2021/05/Manifesto_ENGLISH.pdf.

195 **Soul Quest faced scrutiny from local and federal law:** Joe Mario Pedersen, "DEA Denies Central Florida Church's Request to Use Drug for Religious Purposes," *Orlando Sentinel,* June 23, 2021, https://www.orlandosentinel .com/2021/06/23/dea-denies-central-florida-churchs-request-to-use-drug-for -religious-purposes-report/.

195 **In 2020, Soul Quest sued the DEA:** Griffen Thorne, "How DEA Denies Religious Exemption Petitions," Harris Bricken, February 22, 2022, https://harrisbricken.com/psychlawblog/how-dea-denies-religious-exemption -petitions/.

195 **In a detailed letter denying Soul Quest's exemption request:** William McDermott, letter to Christopher Young, April 16, 2021, https://www.bialabate .net/wp-content/uploads/2021/06/DEA_Denial_Soul_Quest_Exemption_2021 .pdf.

196 **Anthony Coulson, a retired senior DEA agent:** Anthony Coulson, interview with the author, February 3, 2023.

196 **Ian Benouis, an attorney in Texas who advises:** Ian Benouis, interview with the author, July 27, 2022.

201 **Gary joined the Marine Corps in February 1998:** Gary Hess, interview with the author, October 27, 2022.

203 **Joe told me he joined the Marine Corps after a traumatic:** Joe Rovnak, interview with the author, October 25, 2022.

208 **Robert grew up in Barrington, Illinois, a wealthy suburb:** Robert Fitzgerald, interview with the author, October 26, 2022.

12: Reminiscing on My Wars

213 **With our high school graduation a few months away in 1999:** This chapter is largely drawn from the author's recollections.

223 **In the article I wrote about the embed:** Ernesto Londoño, "In Baghdad, a Flimsy Outpost; Members of U.S. Unit, Many Untried, Prepare to Test 'a Good Plan,'" *Washington Post,* March 22, 2007.

224 **In 2017, he died by suicide, according to the *Arizona Republic*:** E. J. Montini, "Montini: Hero Who 'Died' in Iraq, Passes Away Here," *Arizona Republic,* March 18, 2017, https://www.azcentral.com/story/opinion/op

-ed/ej-montini/2017/03/18/montini-iraq-war-brian-scott-mancini-veterans
-administration-suicide/99308428/.

225 **The incentives of those jobs made it easy to get pulled into war:**
Lourdes "Lulu" Garcia-Navarro, interview with the author, February 9, 2023.

228 **The way psychoactive substances like ayahuasca affect memory retrieval:** Manoj Dass, interview with the author, February 8, 2023.

13: A Ketamine "Field Trip"

231 **The psychedelics conference in Miami was fittingly:** Descriptions
and quotes from the conference are drawn from author's observations and
notes.

232 **In 2017, federal regulators designated MDMA:** "FDA Grants Breakthrough Therapy Designation for MDMA-Assisted Therapy for PTSD," MAPS
press release, August 26, 2017, https://maps.org/news/media/press-release-fda
-grants-breakthrough-therapy-designation-for-mdma-assisted-psychotherapy
-for-ptsd-agrees-on-special-protocol-assessment-for-phase-3-trials/.

232 **The following year, the agency granted psilocybin:** "COMPASS Pathways Receives FDA Breakthrough Therapy Designation for Psilocybin Therapy
for Treatment-Resistant Depression," Compass Pathways press release, October 23, 2018, https://www.prnewswire.com/news-releases/compass-pathways
-receives-fda-breakthrough-therapy-designation-for-psilocybin-therapy-for
-treatment-resistant-depression-834088100.html.

233 **Dr. Christopher Pittenger, a psychiatrist who leads:** Christopher Pittenger, interview with the author, November 3, 2022.

233 **Dr. Natalie Gukasyan, a psychiatrist at Johns Hopkins University:**
Natalie Gukasyan, interview with the author, November 3, 2022.

234 **Dr. Michael P. Bogenschutz, a psychiatrist:** Michael P. Bogenschutz,
interview with the author, November 3, 2022.

234 **Janis Phelps, a psychotherapist and professor:** Janis Phelps, interview
with the author, February 24, 2023.

237 **I began contemplating doing a ketamine session:** Ronan Levy, interview with the author, July 26, 2022.

237 **Researchers at Yale University discovered that ketamine provided:**
Jennifer Chen, "Treating Depression: An Expert Discusses Risks, Benefits of

Ketamine," Yale Medicine, October 16, 2017, https://www.yalemedicine.org/news/ketamine-the-new-miracle-drug.

238 But ketamine's patent expired in 2002: "KETAMINE Nomination," NIH, February 13, 2002, https://ntp.niehs.nih.gov/sites/default/files/ntp/htdocs/chem_background/exsumpdf/ketamine_508.pdf.

238 Companies like Field Trip, which is based in Toronto, saw in ketamine: Will Yakowicz, "Field Trip Health, Another Psychedelic Therapy Company, Goes Public," *Forbes*, October 7, 2020, https://www.forbes.com/sites/willyakowicz/2020/10/07/psychedelic-therapy-company-field-trip-health-goes-public-to-revolutionize-mental-health-treatments/?sh=628016ca79a5.

240 "Bring back 'the Happy.' Fast!": Bloom Mental Health, https://www.bloommh.com/ketamine-therapy.html.

241 During our introductory psychotherapy session on a video call: Lauren Cabaldon, interview and sessions with the author, including on November 17, 2022, and February 23, 2023.

14: "Wrecking Ball"

247 Chris Conlogue arrived thirty minutes early: Chris Conlogue, interview with the author, March 11, 2023.

248 The Drug Enforcement Administration lists MDMA: "Ecstasy or MDMA (Also Known as Molly)," DEA, https://www.dea.gov/factsheets/ecstasy-or-mdma-also-known-molly.

249 The MDMA trial at the Loma Linda VA may: Shannon Remick, interview with the author, March 25, 2023.

249 The book was *Food of the Gods*: Terence McKenna, *Food of the Gods: The Search for the Original Tree of Knowledge* (New York: Bantam, 1993).

251 With LSD and psilocybin off the table: "MDMA (Ecstasy) Abuse Research Report," National Institute on Drug Abuse, September 2017, https://nida.nih.gov/publications/research-reports/mdma-ecstasy-abuse/what-is-the-history-of-mdma.

251 It was forgotten until Alexander Shulgin: Udo Benzenhöfer and Torsten Passie, "Rediscovering MDMA (Ecstasy): The Role of the American Chemist Alexander T. Shulgin," *Addiction Journal* 105, no. 8 (August 2010): 1355–61, https://pubmed.ncbi.nlm.nih.gov/20653618/.

251 **MAPS's first major break came in 2001:** Rick Doblin, "A Clinical Plan for MDMA (Ecstasy) in the Treatment of Post-Traumatic Stress Disorder (PTSD): Partnering with the FDA," MAPS, November 2, 2001, https://maps.org/news-letters/v12n3/12305dob.html.

251 **In an interview, Rick told me he came:** Rick Doblin, interview with the author, November 5, 2022.

253 **That raised the possibility of a breakthrough for treating:** Mike Richman, "Study: Economic Burden of PTSD 'Staggering,'" US Department of Veterans Affairs, April 25, 2022, https://www.research.va.gov/currents/0422-Study-economic-burden-of-PTSD-staggering.cfm.

257 **"It was important to us to create a space that didn't":** Allie Kaigle, interview with the author, March 25, 2023.

Epilogue

263 **Bryan began studying psychedelics decades ago:** Bryan Roth, interview with the author, January 18, 2023.

264 **In 2020, the Pentagon awarded Bryan's lab:** "Roth Leads $26.9 Million Project to Create Better Psychiatric Medications," UHC School of Medicine press release, January 15, 2020, https://news.unchealthcare.org/2020/06/roth-leads-26-9-million-project-to-create-better-psychiatric-medications/.

264 **Among its most famous clunkers was:** Duncan Graham-Rowe, "Fifty Years of DARPA: Hits, Misses and Ones to Watch," *New Scientist*, May 15, 2008, https://www.newscientist.com/article/dn13907-fifty-years-of-darpa-hits-misses-and-ones-to-watch/.

264 **Dr. Matthew Pava, the DARPA official who:** Matthew Pava, interview with the author, February 3, 2023.

INDEX

ABOUT THE AUTHOR

Ernesto Londoño is a national correspondent at the *New York Times*, where he has worked since 2014. He was born and raised in Colombia and has spent the past two decades covering some of the most important stories of his generation. He covered the wars in Iraq and Afghanistan and the Arab Spring, served on the editorial board of the *New York Times*, and was the newspaper's bureau chief in Brazil.

CELADON
BOOKS

Founded in 2017, Celadon Books, a division of
Macmillan Publishers, publishes a highly curated list
of twenty to twenty-five new titles a year. The list of
both fiction and nonfiction is eclectic and focuses
on publishing commercial and literary books and
discovering and nurturing talent.